Faith and
the Placebo
Effect

An argument for self-healing

Faith and the Placebo Effect

by

Lolette Kuby

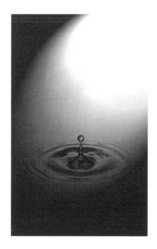

Origin Press
Novato, CA

Origin Press

1122 Grant Ave., Suite C, Novato, CA 94945
888.267.4446 • OriginPress.com

Publisher's Cataloging-in-Publication
(*Provided by Quality Books, Inc.*)

BT
732.5
.K825
2001

Kuby, Lolette,
    Faith and the placebo effect : an argument for
self-healing / Lolette Kuby.—1st ed.
    p. cm.
    Includes bibliographical references.
    LCCN: 2001087711
    ISBN: 1-57983-005-6
    1. Spiritual healing. 2. Mental healing
I. Title.
RZ401.K83 2001   615.8'52
                QB101-200317

Printed in the United States of America
10 9 8 7 6 5 4 3 2 1

To Hally

Contents

Acknowledgements

The birth of a book is a wonderful event. What else, except perhaps the birth of a child, so clearly contains its multiple heritages, and even more than a child, assimilates a web of worldwide and time-defying ideas and influences. A book is indeed a vessel of human unity.

There are so many whom I *should* thank for their ideas and influences that I would need a book for that purpose alone, and there are those whom I must thank: my beloved friends the poet Bonnie Jacobson and psychologists Linda Pendleton and Allen Mumper, who contributed their knowledge and talents and a great deal of their time to fine-combing the early versions of the manuscript—line by line and word by word. Their corrections and suggestions are implanted in this book, and their encouragement helped keep the book alive through multiple drafts. My friends Chrissy Theroux, Judy Churchill, Karl Friedreich, Sherry Jackson, Rita Haulzhausser, and Eddie Muraski acted as first audience, listening attentively and appreciatively through my reading of many chapters.

I need also to acknowledge the librarians at the Mayfield Heights Regional Library in Cleveland, Ohio, for their unusual expertise and helpfulness. And I must express my gratitude to Joan Gattuso, minister of Unity of Greater Cleveland, and her husband, David Alexander, for loving the book and insisting to the universe that it "get out there." I wish to thank my copy editor, Netty Kahan, for her devoted attention to the manuscript and for the sweetness of her disposition. I reserve my special thanks for my publisher and editor, Byron Belitsos, the door through whom this book enters the world, for his unfailing reasonability, his durable patience, for his keen sense of humor, and for having the good sense to be a poet as well as a publisher.

Also, I do not want to neglect to acknowledge the brilliant work of Dr. Howard Brody and Petr Skrabanek, whose ideas and research I drew upon heavily. Although I don't necessarily agree with their conclusions, they fulfill Galen's requirement that "the best physician is also a philosopher, grounded in logic, physics, and ethics." Finally, I also wish to acknowledge my debt to Dr. Oscar Janiger, whose book *A Different Kind of Healing: Doctors Speak Candidly about Their Successes with Alternative Medicine* provided so many testimonies from so many doctors who are beginning to look at the practice of medicine in a different way, and to Leonard White, Bernard Tursky, and Gary E. Schwartz, editors of *Placebo: Theory, Research and Mechanisms,* which contains the most interesting collection of essays on the placebo effect that I have seen gathered into one book.

Faith and
the Placebo
Effect

introduction

Every method of treating illness works. High-tech laboratory-tested therapies of Western medicine work—so do the ancient techniques of Eastern medicine. Laser surgery and chemotherapy, crystals, ginseng root and echinacea bark, low-fat diets and vitamin megadoses, as well as the whole armamentarium of New Age medicine—such as aromatherapy, music therapy, Therapeutic Touch, Reiki, macrobiotics—they all work. Every possible decoction of forest and garden, and yes, a rag, a bone, and a hank of hair have been used to heal and have healed. In the history of the world, there has never been a medicine or a treatment that did not heal someone.

How is this possible? What is really going on here?

To compound the puzzle, why doesn't a given treatment work on everyone who has the same disease? And, if a treatment is effective in Switzerland, why doesn't it work in Swaziland? And, if a treatment worked in the year 1800, why didn't the identical treatment work in the year 1900?

Science always claims to look for the simple answer, the elegant solution. Is there one that could explain this conundrum? Indeed there is. It is the subject of this book.

I am not a doctor or a scientist. I am a poet, a writer, and a professor of English—but one who has experienced profound self-healing. I owe allegiance to no profession, no colleagues, and no industry. I have no educational bias. Indeed, my singular experience demolished my former lifelong bias in favor of medicine and scientific materialism.

Faith and the Placebo Effect is an argument for self-healing. It is also a record of my own mental and spiritual journey. I have assembled ideas from the scriptures and practices of many religions, from philosophers, scientists, doctors, theologians, and from the cultures of many periods and places. I use these plus a wealth of testimonials from ordinary people to make the message carried by the phenomenon of the placebo effect incontrovertible to the thoughtful person. This book is a blend of experience, intuition, research, and mysticism that together form a vision of life and health.

Along with countless others, I have discovered a great truth. Neither I nor the others invented it. The truth is that your health is in your mind.

1

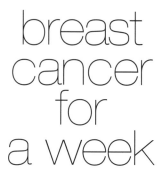

breast
cancer
for
a week

On January 26, 1982, at eight o'clock in the
morning, I entered Cleveland's Suburban Hospital for
a breast augmentation, a simple outpatient procedure,
to be performed by Dr. Sheldon Artz. At two in the afternoon, I exited the hospital with breast cancer. Before Dr.
Artz inserted the silicon implants, he sent to the biopsy
lab a tissue sample of a lump I had asked him to look at
"while I was open." The lab reported back that the lump
was tubular carcinoma of the right breast.[1]

The doctor had tears in his eyes as he stood at my
bedside in the recovery room. He wanted to quickly

schedule me into the hospital for a mastectomy. I'm sure
he expected my immediate panicky acquiescence. I said
no, I had to think. But thinking was the last thing I was
able to do. All my life, cancer had been the one disease
that terrified me. The diagnosis of cancer blew my mind:
It stunned me into a kind of cognitive trance. That afternoon, I was released from the hospital with a sore chest,
the beautiful new 34Bs I had coveted since puberty,
and a vacant mind. It wasn't that I questioned my
former ideas, but that suddenly I had no ideas. As to my
emotions, they consisted of vague, muted fears that
periodically erupted into spurts of panic. Customary patterns of thought could not have been more demolished
if I'd had a lobotomy.

My former husband and all-time friend, Don, who
had chauffeured me to the hospital that morning, drove
me home in stony silence through a typically cold, grey,
Cleveland day. At home, my mental vacuity continued.
In the minute it took for the doctor, who sobbed as he
spoke, to say, "I cut right through it, it's cancer, all for
nothing [the implants], all for nothing!" the world
became meaningless to me. It was as though the world
were a balloon that had been punctured by the word
"cancer." Objects around me had no import, no associa-
tions beyond their literal ones: This was a tea kettle. You
put water into it. You lit a fire under it. When the water
boiled, you poured it over a tea bag. Then you opened
your mouth and drank. This other object was a toilet.
After your body used it, you flushed. The state of my
mind was what Buddhists refer to as "beginners' mind,"
mind dissociated from memory and its judgments, an

amnesia not of facts but of signification.

That evening, Don brought some books and cassette tapes related to religions he labeled "New Thought." For two years he had tried to proselytize me and I had staunchly scoffed at the absurdity of New Thought ideas. Now, he promised they would comfort me, and I was open to any possible source of comfort. I read avidly for the next five days. My mind was no longer blocked by the quick rebuttals of habitual skepticism and cynicism, and what I read amazed and astounded me. Could this be the truth? Was it possible that perfect health could be mine? Was it possible that happiness was my birthright that I had only to claim? Could it be that the ubiquity of God, which Judaism and Christianity had always taught, meant precisely that?—in here, out there, everywhere, without the smallest micrometer of an interstice between me and Him?[2]

Seven days after the surgery, I was certain that these ideas not only were possible, they were the truth of human existence: On the evening of the fifth day, I experienced what I now call a minor revelation, minor only relative to the revelation that occurred on the seventh day (February 1, 1982) at midnight, which no word can name nor tongue utter.

The first revelation brought a vision of Jesus. The second took me into the presence of the Very God. After the revelation, I was not the same person, and I was not my own agent. Reality rearranged itself into a new system, and I was impelled to live my life in a new way. My old eyes had been removed and new ones placed in their sockets. These new eyes saw that the world was not the world I had lived in all my life, but the one described by poets like Gerard Manley Hopkins: "The world is charged with the grandeur of God. It will shine out like shining from shook foil."

For weeks after the revelation, I felt as though my body was surrounded by a silvery aura and that my face shone like Moses' face when he descended from Mt. Sinai. When I looked in the mirror, I saw no aura, but I did see a countenance free of fear, one that, for the first time in my life, I truly liked.

And I knew that I was healed.

For several months I hugged the revelation to my heart as though it were a treasure too precious to share with anyone. Verbalizing would defile it. When I attempted to speak of it, I wept. When finally I told my closest friends, their reaction deeply perplexed and disappointed me. They were more frightened by the cancer than strengthened by the healing, more alarmed by the dreaded disease than awed by the wondrous knowledge I had gained. I thought they would be overwhelmed by the account of my experience and overjoyed because what had happened to me could happen to them—what has been done, can be done. But they doubted the healing or dismissed it as a fortuitous accident. Some doubted the diagnosis of cancer entirely, which of course allowed them to dismiss any idea of healing. One friend did accept the healing as a miracle. But not one of the three "got" what I was telling them about their own extraordinary healing powers.

Five years elapsed before I spoke of my experience again. I realized that in order to convince ordinary people, I needed to find evidence of self-healing grounded in everyday life and unrelated to mysticism. I needed the kind of proof that would appeal to the intelligence of reasonable people. I found that proof in the placebo effect. The placebo effect is the good news of our time: It says, "You have been cured by nothing but yourself."

In its popular definition, the placebo effect means a cure brought about by a medicine or a procedure, say, surgery, that afterward is revealed to be a sham—merely a sugar pill or mock surgery performed with a rubber knife. And that is exactly correct. The placebo effect is an effect with no external cause.

2

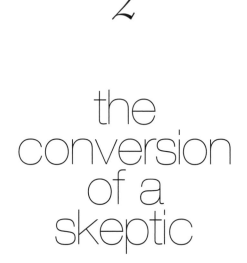

the
conversion
of a
skeptic

*There is no hope for any speculation
that does not look absurd at first glance.*
—*Niels Bohr*

During America's celebration of its one hundredth birthday, a New England newspaper ran an item about a man who was arrested for attempting to obtain money under false pretenses. He claimed he invented a device whereby one person could talk to another several miles away by means of a small apparatus and some wire. Any idea looks ridiculous before its time. In 1492, "they all laughed at Christopher Columbus," as the old Gershwin song says. In 1955, the prospect of a moon walk would have sounded like science fiction to most people.

Since ancient times, medical practitioners have known that sugar pills work. Like everyone else, I had heard accounts of such cures, but, like everyone else, I did not take them seriously. They were curiosities—not applicable to real illness in real life. I certainly didn't want my doctor to give me a sugar pill! I wanted good, sound, state-of-the-art medical treatment that employed all the latest technologies. Like most people, I suspected that if a placebo alleviated a disease, it was because the disease had been "all in the mind" to begin with. Or else I thought it was one of those rare mysterious remissions that certainly no rational person would count on.

As to contemporary faith healers, I believed they were all charlatans of the Elmer Gantry variety, and I believed biblical faith healings were parables or metaphors or exaggerations. To my mind, if you were sick and didn't see a doctor, you were the kind of simpleton who would conduct your life according to the prognostications of astrologers or fortune tellers. When I was a child, there were gypsies living in my neighborhood. Reputed to be thieves and liars, they lived in unoccupied stores and gave readings by crystal ball. At age eight, I felt contempt for anyone who would seek their advice about anything, let alone health matters. When I grew up, I felt a similar disdain for Christian Science; whenever I heard of a Christian Scientist withholding medical treatment from a child, I was just as infuriated as the rest of "rational" society that a helpless innocent suffered

needlessly because of the ignorance or the distorted reli-
giosity of its parents. I believed that all psi phenomena
were trumped up or were illusions that had simple
scientific explanations. In brief, I lumped all things that
could not be explained by the scientific method into a
category labeled "hokum." I was a product of my culture.
Who is not, and how do we become that way?

In my case, I was reared in a family of blue-collar,
Jewish, atheist, old-time Bolsheviks. Religion was a kind
of legerdemain—a sleight of hand that dulled your
reasoning power and diverted your attention from the
deplorable state of your life. It was "the opiate of the
people," the drug with which the rich kept the poor
from rebelling, by promising them pie in the sky in the
hereafter.

But my own personal belief system was dichoto-
mous; for, while my rational mind capitulated to rational
positivism, another part of me, from the time I was a
very little child, secretly believed in God. To accommo-
date this conflict, I described myself as an agnostic.

College didn't alter my cynical worldview, although
my secret belief in God continued. As a literature major
with a minor in philosophy, I was introduced to ideas
that deviated sharply from those of the popular culture,
but these mainly dealt with ethics and aesthetics. My
professors were mostly secular humanists, and if
theories about God and God's relationship with humans
entered the lecture, they entered as intellectual games,
empty abstractions that had no bearing on the real
world.

When I finally got a PhD in English, I still believed

in God, still mostly silently—for no academic mentions God except in the context of literature, history, or anthropology. But what a God I contrived—the fierce, vengeful, proud God of the Old Testament. There are, of course, many aspects of the God of the Old Testament. I chose the one that spent eternity judging the sins of his creation and was most intolerant of the sin of pride. He was the God of the Book of Job—the God who visited destruction upon his servants until they abjectly admitted to knowing nothing. He was the wrathful patriarch of Milton's *Paradise Lost*—the God who brooked no disagreement from even the most favored of his angels. Preeminently he was the God of Melville's Ahab, creator of the killer whale, whom you must thank for taking your leg off lest he retaliate for your thanklessness by taking off the other.

My old God was not implacable. You could change his mind, but you had to beg, cry, implore, promise. You had to make trades: "God, I will not do this if you will not do that." "God, if someone has to have cancer, let it be me instead of my daughter." This God did not emanate love; he doled it out as payment to creatures separate from him—the creation was here, where I am standing, and God was away off there, a Supreme Court judge, untouchable and with lifetime tenure. He was a God of justice—right is right!—so could not desist from killing humans in retribution for their sins unless he supplied his Son to take their suffering upon himself.

It was with this religious disposition that in January of 1982 I entered the hospital for the beautification of my body. As for the events of my life at that time, I had been twice married and divorced, had two grown children, had had an erratic career as an assistant professor of English, a writing consultant and editor, and a director of advertising and public relations. I had been an activist for civil rights, women's rights, and the environment. I loved to have intellectual discussions about God and religion, but I conducted my life as a secular humanist.

I was reasonably healthy. I and my family went to doctors probably less than most: I went for the annual checkup, the pap smear, and the obligatory flu shots when the newspapers warned of still another un-American virus—certainly not for every sniffle or throb. I took vitamins, tried to cut down on junk food, and was fairly physically active—folk dancing, tennis, and heavy gardening. I feared only one disease—cancer. And I feared cancer in only one site—the breast. So, of course, cancer of the breast is what I got. I do not say "of course" ironically; I mean it to be a rational statement. I now fully believe, "What you fear comes upon you."

When the cancer was discovered and my distraught doctor announced that I would need a mastectomy, I replied that what I needed was time to think. By the end of the following week, I was healed. When I returned to the doctor to have the implant stitches removed, he was astonished when I told him that I had decided not to have cancer surgery. The lump in my breast remained, clearly discernible to the touch. Nevertheless I knew that I was cured.

I had the lump surgically removed (for a reason I will explain in chapter 18, "Fighting Disease—A Losing Battle") in 1990, eight years after the original diagnosis.

When the lump was removed I consented to no other treatment—not the conventional lymph node removal, not radiation, and not chemotherapy.

I have never been healthier. Aside from the lumpectomy, I have not visited a doctor since 1982, except for seeing a podiatrist for tennis shoe arch supports.

I know that my healing was not a miracle in the traditional sense. It was a placebo effect—a cure that came about without the employment of any external agency, a miracle that anyone can perform, a self-healing.

If not a miracle, where does God come in? God comes in by any other name—Cosmic Energy, Divine Mind, the Tao, Christ, the Holy Spirit; any name will do that connects the individual with a higher power. Because of my revelation, I know this power to be the Creator God whose universe is perfect and in whose image we are made. But belief in God is not necessary for self-healing. Self-healing is a product of faith, but not necessarily of faith in God.

The response of the medical industry to the placebo effect has been neglect. In 1945, one of the few doctors who investigated the subject was "unable to find any articles on placebos listed in two major medical bibliographic indexes."[3] Now, 50 years later, I find a similar disregard. Organizations like the Institute of Noetic Sciences have looked into the placebo phenomenon, and at the end of the year 2000, the National Institutes of Health finally held a conference on the subject. Yet studies on placebos make up a minute fraction of the huge and continuously burgeoning medical literature. There are other striking omissions. For example, among the hundreds of references on remission that I scanned in preparation of this book, not one had the term "spontaneous remission" in its title. Medical researchers, so zealous in discovering the cause of disease, seem far less interested in cures not attributable to medicine. Yet almost 100 percent of doctors will concede that disease, including cancer, does unaccountably disappear. Few doctors have the courage to openly admit that *80 percent* of illnesses will heal themselves. The great majority of doctors simply ignore earthshaking statements that challenge the profession, even when those statements come from someone high in their own ranks such as Sir Douglas Black, a past president of Britain's Royal College of Physicians, who claims that modern medical treatment affects the outcome of only 10 percent of diseases.[4]

One of the few investigators into the placebo phenomenon, Dr. H.K. Beecher, found that almost 40 percent of the hundreds of patients he tested benefited from placebos. He points out that placebos "have been given credit for almost all medical cures throughout history," and that placebos "must be the single most effective medicine known to man."[5] Yes—the sugar pill is the philosophers' stone sought by alchemists throughout the ages.

Yet these startling statements hardly budge the medical mindset. "Noncauses" of cures remain a mystery that the medical industry scarcely explores.

In my own case, neither the doctor who originally verified the presence of cancer cells, nor the one who did the lumpectomy eight years later, showed any interest in my continued health. My self-healing, to the extent they were willing to believe it, made me an eccentric, like a flagpole sitter or goldfish swallower.

"Well, I guess your magic is stronger than my magic," said Dr. Artz.

"I can't force you to take the usual treatments because yours is not the usual case. Most people aren't as lucky as you," said Dr. Levy.

They did not ask what might be behind my "magic" or my "luck." They did not ask what I was eating, drinking, thinking, or feeling. Here I was, a person with a verified cancer, who agreed to none of the traditional treatments, and I was stating that I never felt better. Wouldn't you think the doctors would be curious? Wouldn't you think they might ask me to participate in a study of anomalous cases? To my knowledge, no comprehensive study exists of people who have had a serious ailment that mysteriously disappeared.

If someone's cancer is not medically treated, that person does not enter the statistics on cancer. The statistics therefore are completely skewed in favor of conventional treatment by chemotherapy, radiation, and other damaging procedures. People who either do not visit doctors for a diagnosis or do not follow up with medical treatment for a diagnosed disease simply do not show up in the data.

The placebo effect has been recognized by that rubric for hundreds of years. It has also been named miracle, magic, hex, and voodoo. Whatever it is called, it is the most obvious, most universal, and oldest proof we have that what cures human beings is not an external agent, but their own mind. By *mind* I do not mean the rational faculty. I mean the totality of brain, feelings, senses, unconscious and conscious awareness, intuition, soul, spirit, and all else unnamed that constitutes consciousness.

It took ten years of formal education to get my PhD It has taken me several years longer than that to gain the insights and acquire the information and hearken to the divine guidance that enables me to make this claim: If you have had an idea that you have assimilated deeply, so deeply that it is no longer an idea but part of the very structure of your consciousness, then what was once an idea is now your faith. The placebo effect comes into play when an idea concerning your health has become your faith. Anything can function as a placebo; chemotherapy and sugar pills function in exactly the same way.

3

miracle
or mind?

Miracles do not happen in contradiction to nature,
but only in contradiction to what is known to us of nature.

—*St. Augustine*

You do not have to know what the sun is made
of to see by its light. You do not have to understand
electricity to flick on a switch, nor understand brain
chemistry to think. And you do not have to investigate
the etiology of any disease or any given treatment in
order to experience the placebo effect.

What exactly is a placebo effect? In the first chapter
I defined it as an effect with no external cause. This
sounds like a paradox; the absence of cause would
logically preclude the possibility of effect. But what
seems to be paradoxical may simply indicate that we
have stumbled across the edge of our ignorance: Paradox

marks a limitation of knowledge, not an impossibility in reality. Much of modern physics is defined by apparent paradox. Physicists investigate whether light is composed of waves or particles, that is, of energy or matter, and the answer they receive is, paradoxically, both.[6] The paradox of the placebo effect is far easier to resolve: It is the external effect of an internal cause. That is, it is a physical demonstration of a state of mind.

Doctors have attempted to define the placebo effect, but very few are as willing as Dr. Douglas Black, the aforementioned president of Britain's College of Physicians, to pull the rug out from under the whole medical profession. Dr. Black said, "New drugs create new hopes," and he advised an audience of doctors that "one should treat as many patients as possible with a new drug *while it still has the power to heal.*"[7] (Italics mine.) The implications should have boggled the minds of the audience: Why would a patient's hope increase the power of a pharmacological substance, and what could cause such a substance to lose its power? But physicians' responses to statements such as Dr. Black's reminds me of the humorous TV commercial in which two men lost in the desert stumble right past the Land Rover that could carry them to safety, because they think it is a mirage.

The word "placebo" can be traced back to the four-teenth century when it was used in vespers chanted for the dead, and derives from the Latin translation of Psalm 116.9: "Placebo Domino in regione vivorum" [I will please the Lord in the land of the living]. Placebo came to mean "I shall please"; but today its usual connotation is to please by deception. *Hooper's Medical Dictionary* of 1811 defined placebo as "an epithet given to any medi-cine adopted to please rather than to benefit the patient." A hundred and eighty-two years later, in 1993, *Merriam-Webster's Collegiate Dictionary*, 10th Edition, defines it almost the same way: "a medication prescribed more for the mental relief of the patient than for its actual effect on a disorder." A 1973 edition of *The Dictionary of Behavioral Science* (DBS) begins with a more promising definition: "a substance with no medicinal properties which causes a patient to improve because of his belief in its efficacy." But the DBS goes on to negate the idea that real improve-ment occurs: "It reinforces the patient's expectations though it *does not really act on the individual's condition*." (Italics mine.)

The usual definitions of the placebo effect imply fakery and reinforce commonplace assumptions like these: (1) If a patient responds to a placebo, his symptom was either feigned or imaginary. (2) The only symptoms placebos can act upon are anxiety or pain. (3) Placebos, whether they help or not, at least are harmless. (4) Only neurotic personality types respond to placebos.

Psychologists and psychiatrists are the two cate-gories of health professionals that show the most interest in the placebo effect, and each school of psychotherapy contributes its own spin.

Behavioral psychology finds the placebo effect akin to the Pavlovian response: Just as a dog salivates when a bell associated with food rings, so a patient enters a cure mode when something associated with a cure is present. The conditioning agent need not be medicine: It could be the setting—a doctor's office or a hospital—where one expects to get help. It could be merely attention from a surrogate of the person who in the patient's childhood "kissed it and made it better"—a role most often played by a doctor. Behavioral psychologists have indeed come close to the truth of self-healing. They recognize the power of association and expectation to function as placebos, yet they refrain from articulating the conclusion that the psyche governs healing.

Among psychotherapists in general there is much grappling with the definition. A placebo has been called all of the following:

1. any nonspecific treatment

2. anything nonintentional in the treatment

3. anything incidental to the treatment

4. anything deliberately used that the doctor believes to be ineffective or pharmacologically inert

5. any pharmacologically active substance that brings about a completely unaccountable result

6. variables that accompany any treatment that are considered to be irrelevant to the treatment

7. the belief of the patient that he or she is in a healing context

Taken together these definitions broaden the concept of placebo to include everything—real medicines and sugar pills, voodoo dolls and physician's personalities, surgery and a good day at work, a doctor's office and the shrine at Lourdes. And a placebo effect would include not only good effects but also bad effects.[8]

This is exactly right. In other words, the number of placebos is infinite. A placebo may be anything—intended and not intended, an active and an inert drug, the disposition of the doctor and the faith of the patient. Any of these may trigger a cure or may intensify an illness.

Now we are in territory where science as currently practiced cannot go, for science seeks to pinpoint the exact cause of any given effect: It simply can't handle a phenomenon that can be caused by anything and that may be equally not caused by the same "anything." We are in metaphysical territory, the territory of the mind.

4

the evidence

*Any idea seriously entertained tends to bring about
the realization of itself.*

—*Joseph Chilton Pearce*

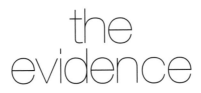

When my own healing occurred, I knew that I was
cured of cancer, but I didn't understand why or how. I
was tempted to call the cure a miracle, but I rejected that
idea. For what a grandiose event a miracle is; how it
elevates the recipient! A miracle would have meant that
God had chosen me above so many others. I couldn't kid
myself that I was more deserving: I was no smarter, no
kinder, no more talented, no more of anything. Was
God, then, capricious? Did he draw lottery numbers?
Did he favor blue eyes and brown hair? The more I

investigated, the more clear it became that my healing was only one among uncountable others.

In everyday life, unexplained healings happen all the time. Doctors shrug them off or call them "spontaneous remissions," which is simply another way of saying, "We don't have a clue." If the term "placebo effect" is used, it is a derisive catchall that means, "not important enough to take seriously." One doctor's comment is typical: Upon hearing that many people swear by the curative properties of the plant "skullcap," the doctor responded, "That a nearly worthless and essentially inactive plant material could be recommended as a useful tranquilizing herb and praised as an excellent herb for almost any nervous system malfunction says much about the gullibility of human beings."[9] The doctor doesn't deny that people believe they have in fact benefited from skullcap; yet, having decided that the "worthless plant" can't be the source of the benefit, he fails to ask himself what then the source might be. What is the connection, he might wonder, between gullibility and the apparent power of the plant?

Placebos are of course used in double-blind and even triple-blind studies as controls to test new drugs. A drug's effectiveness is called into question when a placebo produces identical results, as it often does. Pharmaceutical companies then adjust the composition of the drug. But they disregard entirely the obvious puzzle: How can sugar water produce the same effect as a pharmacologically active substance? The aim of "blind" studies is to find a drug that works better than a placebo.

The truly urgent questions should be why a placebo works at all. In the same vein, doctors disregard the implication when a treatment they have been using *successfully* for years proves, with further research, to be totally valueless.

One issue related to placebos that many doctors do take seriously is whether or not administering placebos is ethical. In research, is it ethical to withhold a certain drug from a control group in order to test its effect on another group? In private practice, is it ethical to prescribe salt water with a fancy name? The moral debate goes back centuries. In the eighteenth century, Dr. Samuel Johnson argued against using placebos: "Deception would inevitably prove a noxious instance of disrespect." In the nineteenth century, Oliver Wendell Holmes argued in favor of them: "Your patient has no more right to all the truth you know than he has to all the medicines in your saddlebags." A practical moralist might point out that if placebos are purposely given and the patient finds out that the prescribed medication wasn't "real," he or she would lose faith in the doctor. The irony of this objection is that the *doctor* is a placebo, too; many feel better simply because of their faith in the doctor's power to cure them.

Often, especially in former times, patients have not been told that a placebo was administered, that they had been cured by "nothing," that what the patient believed to be a powerful drug, an injection, or a surgical procedure was actually a bread pill, a syringe filled with distilled water, or a rubber knife. Once in my life that I know of, I was the subject of a placebo experiment, and the experimenter, a dentist, did tell me the truth. I used to be the kind of person who felt pain just by looking at the dentist drill hanging over my head. A shot of Novocain in the jaw wasn't pleasant but at least it was quick. This time, instead of using Novocain, the dentist told me that there was a brand-new painkilling salve. The dentist rubbed some of the Vaseline-like substance on my gum and, after waiting a minute or two, proceeded to drill. "Any pain?" he asked. "No," I replied. So he went on drilling and filling, and I was delighted that I wouldn't be numb and lopsided for the next few hours. Afterward he admitted that the salve was a placebo. At the time, I found this to be nothing but an interesting curiosity. For the doctor, it probably confirmed that the placebo effect could occur in dentistry. To my knowledge, he did not investigate further into the reason the application of "nothing" could prevent pain.

Consensus in the ethics debate holds that it is unethical to administer placebos. Of course, the entire argument would be moot if placebos did not work. But isn't it the farther reaches of absurdity to argue about the ethics of using something that works—just because it is not a medicine?

That voodoo chants can remove disease, or that crystals can eliminate a migraine headache, that tribal drumming can increase fertility, that the water of holy wells or the shrine at Lourdes can mend the lame, or that astrology can forecast tomorrow's events—these are seen as miracles by religious people, available to only a mysteriously elected few. To "rational" people they're nothing but superstitions. I am both a religious and a rational person, and I too dismiss the idea that beating on a drum can induce conception, or that removing needles from a clay doll can bring health. But I cannot dismiss the reality of the outcome: The woman does get pregnant; the man's fever does subside; the cancer is cured by a dip into the Jordan River.

Certainly, not all scientists are willing to simply ignore mysterious cures. Instead they look for "scientific" answers. One doctor, who could not deny the benefits of certain waters and fountains deemed holy, finds that "holiness" is actually an unusual combination of chemicals. He explains, "Wells and springs were believed to have curative qualities because some saint has passed over the stream. . . . The waters in pagan times were consecrated to the Gods." These superstitions, he says, "prevented the medicinal value of the water from being recognized for what it really was."[10]

But this scientific explanation is as problematic as the religious one. The streams and fountains this doctor refers to are found around the globe. Surely they do not all possess identical chemical properties. You would expect a scientist to look for the common denominator of a widespread phenomenon. If the common denominator is not the chemistry of the far-flung waters, and if it is not the influence of a Christian saint or pagan god, might it not be the faith of the people who bathe in the waters?

Medical literature is replete with accounts of mysterious effects, both beneficent and evil. For each one recorded there must be thousands of others. Here are some samples:

In 1916, a woman named Joan Flower, who *believed herself to be a witch* but wanted to escape punishment, swallowed a mouthful of bread and butter, declaring her wish that it might never go through her if she were guilty. She dropped dead on the spot.[11]

The book *The Remains of Denis Granville* gives an account of a Frenchman suffering from melancholia (now called depression or affective disorder). While a priest prayed, a surgeon made a small incision in the sick man's side, and at the same time a physician suddenly released a bat from a bag. Convinced that the bat was an evil spirit that had left his body through the cut, the patient made an instant recovery.[12]

In Mexico, a terrible epidemic followed upon a belief that witches and wizards possessed the power to leave their own bodies and enter other people. Many who walked out at night believed they had been attacked by these disincarnate sorcerers and quickly faded into illness and death.[13]

We are inclined to read these accounts in the same spirit as we read science fiction. But are they any more strange than the dichotomies in the health of a person suffering from multiple personality disorder? One of the multiple "selves" may have a medically verified allergy or dermatitis, while another of the "selves" is completely free of these ailments. The same body produces both these physical states on cue, depending upon which personality is in control!

Are they any more strange than the fact that a person with a missing limb can feel an itch in that limb, and can relieve the itch by scratching air?

Are they any more strange than that a woman vomits *before* she goes in for chemotherapy? Her vomiting is real, yet nothing has been done to the woman to induce severe nausea. Could whatever causes the vomiting be the same thing that caused the cancer to begin with?

And isn't it strange that a particular disease can be cured in different societies using entirely different treatments?—or that the same disease would not be cured within the same society by different doctors using the same treatment?

It stretches credulity to think that people with particular illnesses coincidentally congregate in one place. Yet medical records of one town show double the number of tonsillectomies or gall bladder removals or mastectomies as that of another town: "It is not unusual for doctors in one community to perform hysterectomies, say, at two or three times the rate of doctors in another town. Rates for some cardiac procedures differ around the country by as much as 50 percent."[14] What accounts for this differential popularity of certain surgical procedures? The perceived need is "in the air," so to speak, not carried by virus or bacteria, but by mental contagion. Evidence does show that people cope or recover or even die, depending not upon the virulence of the illness but upon the vision of the disease held by their doctors.

Medicine is supposed to rest on scientific objectivity. If you bump into an organism that causes smallpox, you are supposed to get smallpox, not cholera. Yet there does seem to be such a thing as disease selectivity. The same "cause," for example, a deficiency of vitamin C, will lead to gum disease in one person, frequent colds in another. The consumption of fatty foods will cause one person to develop clogged arteries, another gall bladder disease. Of four people subjected to intensely stressful situations, one might select to have an ulcer, another a stiff neck, another cancer, and the fourth nothing. People are also "treatment selective." For any group of ulcer patients, for example, a pill might work on one, an herb on another, massage on another, and surgery on another. One might try to account for disease selectivity on the basis of biochemical individuality, organic weakness, coincidence, or genetic structure, but none of these can be conclusively proven to be the cause of a specific disease in a specific individual. I know that I selected cancer of the breast out of a world of potential diseases because it corresponded to my own subconscious need. I submit that the selection of the treatment and the selection of the ailment point to the attitudes and beliefs of the patient rather than to objective causes and cures of disease.

Heart problems, for example, are low in Japan. Arthritis is low among the Hunza. Research looks for dietary or lifestyle correlations: The Japanese have healthy hearts because they don't eat much meat, or because they eat a lot of rice, or because their diet is low in fat. The Hunza don't get arthritis because they eat yogurt and do demanding physical work. But then it is found that the French and Italian heart disease rate is also low, yet the culinary tastes of both countries lean strongly to meat and cheese. Forced to come up with another "scientific" answer, it is now explained that red wine—the favored beverage of both countries—counteracts the deleterious effect of meat and that fermented fat, for example, cheese, is not cholesterol forming. But if diet or exercise is the explanation, how does it happen that when Japanese come to America and become bombarded like the rest of us with fearsome information about heart disease they begin to experience just as much heart trouble as the rest of us, *even those Japanese who continue to adhere to their ancestral diet*?

Not only do we get the ills and cures we expect to get, we can even fend off death until we're ready. In China few old women die *during* the festival of O-bon, and many die immediately afterward.[15] In Israel, far fewer people died during two doctors' strikes (many years apart) than immediately afterward. It is as though someone gave those people a magic pill that would prevent dying until they themselves found the time more propitious.

Most physicians would agree that "prior to the advent of scientific medicine near the turn of the twentieth century, most remedies administered by physicians had little or no curative power."[16] Yet people throughout the ages have in fact been cured by these remedies—remedies that today are *known* to possess no curative power.

Up until about one hundred years ago, the greatest causes of death were accident (including natural catastrophe and war), infectious diseases, and travails of childbirth. The entire array of physical problems about which people now consult doctors were formerly cured by methods and medicines now considered worthless. Yet these methods and medicines alleviated symptoms just as do our modern treatments. One often-quoted expert of our time writes, "Since almost all medications until recently were placebos, the history of medical treatment can be characterized largely as the history of the placebo effect."[17]

Go back two hundred years and you will hear Thomas Jefferson say, "One of the most successful physicians I have ever known has assured me that he used more of bread pills, drops of colored water, and powders of hickory ashes, than of all other medicines put together." Note that this doctor was successful. His patients were not dropping like swatted flies.

Go back to 1628 and hear Robert Burton, physician and author of *The Anatomy of Melancholy*, say, "Required in a patient is confidence, to be of good cheer, and have sure hope that his Physician can help him. . . . Otherwise his Physick will not be effectual."

Go back to the Renaissance and hear the great essayist Montaigne say, "For what reason do doctors arouse the credulity of their patients with false promises of cure other than to make their fraudulent nostrums work through the effects of the imagination. . . . One of the masters of their trade has written that there are people for whom the mere sight of a medicine effects a cure."

Physicians throughout the ages have built their

reputations on the placebo effect. One study shows that placebos are 60 percent as effective as the "real" pain-killers, aspirin and morphine.[18] It is very rare for a medicine to have an effective rate higher than 60 percent, even by its manufacturer's claims.

In recent years, articles on the placebo effect, rare as they are, have come from widely diverse areas—Britain, Canada, Spain, France, and South Africa. And they have come from various fields of study—geriatrics, dentistry, psychiatry, allergy and immunology, and surgery. A few courageous, wise doctors and scientists do speak out. One of them admits, "Many papers have demonstrated the importance and magnitude of the placebo effect in every therapeutic area. Placebos can be more powerful than, and reverse the action of, potent active drugs. The incidence of placebo reactions approaches 100 percent in some studies. Placebos can have profound effects on organic illnesses, including incurable malignancies."[19]

The same researcher points to studies that show that placebos "modify both subjectively reported and objectively observable symptoms."[20] They can produce relief of cough, mood swings, angina pectoris, headache, seasickness, anxiety, hypertension, depression, and the common cold. They can lower blood sugar in diabetics and shrink tumors in patients with lymphosarcoma.

That isn't all. Placebos, like drugs, can produce negative side effects—somnolence, palpitations, irritability, insomnia, weakness, a drop in blood pressure, temporal headache, diarrhea, and itching. One study reports that after taking an inert placebo, a patient developed a florid rash that a dermatologist diagnosed as a classic drug-induced dermatitis. In another study, 56 students were given either a pink sugar pill that they were told was a stimulant or a blue sugar pill that they were told was a sedative. Thirty-two percent of those who took the "stimulant" pills said they felt less tired. Those who took the "sedative" pills felt drowsy, and felt more drowsy if they took two. One-third of the total reported undesirable side effects including headaches, dizziness, watery eyes, staggering gait, and abdominal discomfort. Only three reported that the pills had no effect.[21]

Placebos in the guise of medicine mimic drugs in every possible way: the lapse of time between administration and peak effect; the cumulative symptom relief over time; and the carry-over effect after the placebo is stopped. As with drugs, a placebo capsule is more powerful than a placebo pill; an injection works better than either; and an injection that stings works better than a painless one.[22] Placebo surgery is especially powerful. Mock surgery can work just as well as actual surgery, and surgery that has no relationship with the ailment has restored a patient to health.[23]

Placebos are so powerful that the moral issue may not be pertinent, for it seems that patients experience benefits even when the doctor confesses ahead of time that the medication is a placebo. Fourteen outpatients with neurotic complaints participated in a study in which the doctor admitted he was using a sugar pill but said that others had benefited from it. Some of the patients thought the doctor was fooling them and that it was actually a real drug. Some believed it was a sugar pill but said that it helped by making them aware of their own ability to cope. Every one of the patients benefited from a pill they knew was a placebo![24]

Some would regard this study as flawed because the patients' desire to please the doctor may account for their improvement. But, of course, improvement for no reason other than one's desire to please the doctor is itself a placebo effect.

As would be expected, studies have been conducted to try to determine whether some people are placebo "reactor types," and if so, whether they are perhaps weaker willed than other people, more suggestible, passive, and vulnerable to manipulation. The findings were contradictory and confusing to an extent permitting only one conclusion: People who responded to placebos were no more and no less happy, no more and no less neurotic, and no more and no less introverted than the general population.[25]

If it is true that in every way placebos mimic "active" drugs and intentional treatments, isn't it reasonable to ask whether the placebo produces a drug effect or whether the drug produces a placebo effect? Instead of controlling to eliminate the placebo effect, I should think that medical experiments would attempt to reproduce it. But who would be interested in doing that? That kind of experiment would yield far less monetary reward than the profits now enjoyed by pharmaceutical companies and conventional medicine. Drug companies spend millions in controlled studies of a single drug, which, released to the marketplace, brings them more millions. But who would investigate the efficacy of hexes or crystals or injections of water when very little money would follow a positive finding? Indeed, huge profits would be lost if it turned out that a placebo alleviated a given symptom as effectively as a drug.

Putting aside the issue of profits, research may be lacking because in one sense the placebo effect is resistant to scientific inquiry. I already mentioned some nonmedical causes of disease and health. I can mention many more. Sickness, including chronic sickness, and death increase sharply in periods of severe economic fluctuation—whether it be prosperity or recession. We can postulate all sorts of reasons for this coincidence: During recessions, too little nutritious food is eaten; in prosperous periods, too much rich food is eaten. During recessions, people worry about making money; in prosperous periods, they worry about losing it.

Also, as practically everyone by now acknowledges, stress and anxiety cause illness, whatever the cause of the stress and anxiety—losing a job, starting a job, separating from a spouse, moving to another city, marrying early, marrying late, having children, not having children. Conversely, stability and good relationships at home and at work promote health. By implication we can add practically anything to this list of nonmedical factors that promote well- or ill-being: rapport with the doctor, a traffic jam, the patient's conviction that a certain drug works, a frightening news broadcast, and the elation or dejection that accompany high or low golf scores.

The fact is, on any given day for any given individual, the number of things that can influence feelings of well- or ill-being, health and illness, are infinite. The *sine qua non* of scientific investigation is to establish the boundaries that control variables. But the variables that produce placebo effects cannot be controlled.

Double-blind scientific experiments establish three groups: one that receives the active treatment, one that believes it is receiving the active treatment but receives a placebo, and one that receives neither. In more sophisti- cated triple-blind experiments, the doctor is also kept "blind" because it has been found that the doctor's own expectations transfer subconsciously to the patients. To conduct research into the operation of placebos, a fourth control group would have to be included—a group com- posed of people who had not sought a doctor's advice and did not know they were participating in an experi- ment, and they would need to be handled by a doctor who did not know he was handling a group. This fourth group would be essential in order to rule out (1) the effect that comes into play merely from participating in an experiment (the Hawthorne effect) and (2) the expec- tations of people who go to doctors because they believe themselves to be sick.

The absence of research on causeless cures seriously flaws conclusions about health and disease. I claim that people by the millions are cured of illnesses doctors never see. Can this be proven in a laboratory or by statis- tical tables that take no account of people like me who don't go to doctors? How is it possible to determine that a placebo effect has taken place when none has been administered purposely?

The placebo effect rests on anecdotal evidence, and such evidence is widespread beyond calculation. It is replicated and replicable, only not in the laboratory, for the multitudinous variables cannot be controlled. I will note again, as others have, that the greater the ability to limit variables and thereby control the experiment, the less the experiment duplicates life. Science does not own empirical evidence. Your experience and mine are as empirical as you can get. As one doctor put it, the placebo effect is "universal and most likely common in all events of human pathology and healing."[26]

Yes, it happens constantly. If you continue to protest that the effect is all in the mind, meaning that the patient who becomes sleepy after taking a placebo sleeping pill is not really sleepy but only thinks he is, or that the patient who vomits after taking a placebo "drug" only thinks she is nauseated, my answer is: "Of course—the placebo effect is all in the mind!"

5

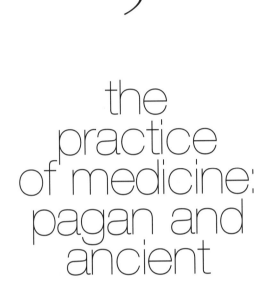

the practice of medicine: pagan and ancient

Faith in the healing power of a dead sardine's head would make it heal.

—*Japanese proverb*

When the plastic surgeon who discovered the cancer during a routine breast augmentation appeared in a state of extreme agitation at my bedside and cried, "I cut right through it!" he expected me to concur (as any "rational" woman would) with the desperate haste of his plan to schedule me for a mastectomy. My amazing calm (spurts of panic came later) may have been psychic numbness or residual anesthetic, but I now think that a deep undercurrent faith was already taking part in my recovery. At any rate, I told the doctor I needed time to think.

By the time I returned to his office to have the stitches removed, he had mailed back to me the sizable fee I had paid him for the augmentation, with a note saying I would need the money for surgery. During my visit, he asked what I had decided, and I replied I was still thinking. But I knew in my heart that I was cured and that I would do what the medical profession would call "nothing."

When I saw him for the routine two-week follow-up, looking very robust and healthy, he asked again about the mastectomy.

My answer stunned him. "Aren't you going to do anything about the cancer?"

"I *am* doing something," I said. I proceeded to offer the details he would be likely to understand: "I've stopped smoking and I'm exercising and eating more healthfully." Then I added the important part: "And I'm doing some spiritual work. I guess *you* would call it praying."

"Well," he replied offhandedly, "your magic is stronger than my magic."

Obviously, his words carried no real significance for him; he inquired no further into what this spiritual work, my "magic," might be.

"Your magic is stronger than my magic." The doctor spoke far better than he knew.

Magic has cured disease and caused it, killed and delivered from death since time immemorial. Shamans of primitive societies used magic; physicians of the ancient world used magic; even Jesus used the techniques and devices magicians used.

All primitive societies[27] recognize some of their members as being supernaturally endowed with the power to cure or kill—we call them witch doctors. They are the ones who possess the occult formula, the secret combination of materials and words with which they can perform superhuman feats: They can induce fertility, impotence, or barrenness; reverse conditions of prosperity or poverty; and arouse love or loathing. Their medicines might be excrement, spittle, leaves, roots, berries, stones, twigs, or water—practically every element in nature. With these they cure boils, stomach pains, warts, tumors, convulsions, and catatonia—practically every ailment in nature. A witch doctor's concoction might consist of dog hair, the roots of a stinkweed plant, and dust scraped from a pink stone. This he or she might fling in the air or bury in the ground, or toss on a fire, while talking in some mysterious language. That both cures and illnesses (even illness unto death) result from such weird procedures is well documented by anthropologists.

Evidence of magical thinking is found in the

dimmest recesses of the human record. The famous cave drawings that show slain animals and victorious hunters seem to have been a kind of mimetic magic enabling the hunter to gain power over his quarry. Primitive societies, even today, ensure the success of a hunt by first acting out the movements of the pursuit in a ritual dance. Could practices such as drawing pictures or dancing cause anything to happen? Reason of course says no. Dancing around a pretend animal cannot possibly bring the real animal to the point of the hunter's spear. Yet, imagine what a different hunting party it would be if, instead of acting out victory, the hunters anticipated failure and spent the day before the hunt worrying about returning empty-handed. Magical thinking changes nothing but the minds of the hunters, and in doing so, it changes the result of the hunt as surely as if it put a spell on the hunted animals.

Ancient Greece, Egypt, and Israel had "witch doctors" of their own kind—an elect few who were believed to be endowed by the gods with the power to heal. It was supposed that physicians were able to read the secrets of the universe, hidden in every natural object and in every human gesture. They were attuned to the occult significance of sneezing, blinking, pointing, spitting, shouting, weeping, whistling, dancing, playing, eating and drinking, defecating, and engaging in sexual intercourse. Sometimes exceptional healers were themselves elevated to the status of a god. The physician Aesculapius, for example, was deified by the Greeks. Thrita was honored in the same way by the Persians, and Dhan-Wantari by the Hindus.[28]

Persia recognized three categories of doctors. Surgeons, or the "knife doctors," occupied the lowest rung of the medical ladder. Next came the "herb doctors." The highest were the true magicians, the "word doctors," who treated the sick only with signs and incantations: "For he will drive away sickness from the body of the faithful"—perhaps vehemently chanting a spell like Bar Bazia, Mas Masia, Kas Kasia, Sharlai and Amarlai!

I doubt that my breast surgeon meant by my "magic" that I was engaged in weird rituals. But something had driven sickness from my body. And something has healed all the generations of humanity before the arrival of "scientific" medicine. If that something is not demons and beneficent spirits and magical words and concoctions, what is it?

I maintain that disease is caused by demons, now as it was then. Disease generates in the "hell" that the poet John Milton located as "you yourself." The habitat of demons is the psyche of the individual, now as it was then. It is no more effective to throw modern drugs at diseases than it is to ring bells to scare them away.

Let me relate a few more of the medical practices found in ancient civilization, the Old Testament, the Gospels, and early Christianity—practices that cannot be understood except as placebos.

In the early days of the tribes of Israel, certain objects were thought to have the power to ward off demons. Individuals made their own decisions about which objects were so endowed, just as today any child can believe that a certain stone or marble is "lucky." Later, the decision was taken out of the individual's hands and the rabbis required "replication": three approved persons had to test the effectiveness of the object in at least three cases before it could rank as a talisman or amulet.[29] As a rule, the rabbis and Jesus abjured magic, yet the Bible contains many accounts of magical practices. The magi who followed the star of Bethlehem to Jesus' birthplace, were of course magicians. And Jesus himself was thought to be a magician. Like the rabbis, he stressed that healing came directly from God. But at various times he used the devices of the magicians: his own spittle, a handful of earth, and words uttered with great vehemence—"Abatha! Come forth!" In biblical times, exactly as in present-day voodoo and aboriginal societies, articles belonging to a person, or sloughs from a person's body—hair, nail clippings, urine—were believed to bear the person's qualities, which could be transferred to others. Paul's clothing was placed on the sick and "the diseases departed from them." When Peter walked by, the sick were brought on cots out into the thoroughfare so that his healing shadow might fall on them.[30]

A hundred years after Jesus, the greatest of Greek physicians, Galen, taught his disciples to accept the possibility of miraculous cures. And he advised his patients to obey any instructions they received in a vision.

Toward the end of the fourth century, the Christian emperor Theodosius, attempting to destroy the magical practices of paganism, demolished the temples where the non-Christian physicians practiced. But magic assumed a Christian coloration and continued. Instead of attaching a separate god to this or that geographical location, Christianity attached a separate saint. Instead of assigning responsibility for various bodily parts to signs of the zodiac, Christianity again substituted saints. For example, St. Otillia is ruler over the head; St. Blasus, over the neck.

If we could stand back and objectively view contemporary medical practices, they would seem as bizarre as some of the treatments practiced in primitive and ancient societies. Today, if a person is distressed by an internal organ, say the gallbladder, his body is opened and the organ is cut out. If a person has a tumorous growth, a deadly poison is dripped into his veins. If a person is sexually debilitated, he could go to a clinic in Great Britain for an injection of pig embryo or horse blood. If a man feels lethargic or low on élan vital, he could be rejuvenated by having his sperm ducts blocked. In fact, in 1911 in Austria, a hundred teachers and university professors—including Sigmund Freud and the great Irish poet W.B. Yeats—did exactly that.[31]

The history of medicine, both ancient and modern, is replete with the logical fallacy called *post hoc ergo propter hoc* (translated as "it comes after, therefore it is caused by"). If a treatment is given—say, radiation or the release of bats from a bag—and the patient gets better, must we assume strict cause and effect? Yet, muses one doctor, "Such is the need of both patients and doctors to believe in treatment that this assumption is widespread and is a potent cause of delusion."[32]

We may strongly suspect that injections of pig embryo cells don't enable erections, that vasectomies don't restore libido, and that Peter's shadow didn't cure scurvy or scrofula. Yet people have sworn that they enjoyed these benefits.

What I have given in this chapter is not a glimpse of the history of medicine, but a glimpse of the history of the placebo effect—effect with no external cause.

6

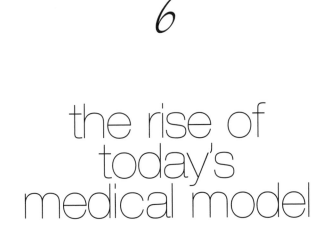

the rise of today's medical model

Premum nil nocere: First do no harm.
—*Hippocrates*

I used to be a confirmed believer in the annual
checkup. Every year, a gynecologist addressed my pelvic
and breast areas (pap smear and mammogram), and a
general practitioner attended the rest of me. I didn't need
the least sign of a physical problem to schedule this
annual checkup. I could be in the pink of condition,
yet not feel secure in my health until a doctor assured
me I was okay. My health belonged to the physician; I
couldn't claim it until the doctor granted me "a clean bill
of health."

The rationale for seeing a doctor when nothing is wrong is "early detection." Our organs, our blood, our brain could be secretly harboring an enemy, a sinister invader who might already be scaling our ramparts. Nemesis awaits our procrastination of the yearly exam. If 13 months go by, during the 13th month we are filled with anxiety. Aside from the wasted money and time, and aside from the actual damage that could be caused by "early detection" (more on this later), routine examination puts us at odds with our own body. Dire warnings issued by health institutions bombard us with the catastrophic consequences that await us if we miss a minuscule sign of the "enemy."

We are, in fact, terrified by illness and convinced of our own inadequacy to treat it, a combination that gives great power to healers of every stripe—shamans, witch doctors, physician-priests—and to none more than to the modern MD. We feel that our bodies belong to us in much the same way that a car or a washing machine belongs to us: And how many of us know how to repair an electrical system or an engine?

Ironically, premodern physicians were expected to possess far more impressive credentials than ours today carry. In primitive societies, tribal healers often earned their elevated status by miraculously overcoming some crippling debility of their own, such as lameness or blindness. They were physicians who literally demonstrated the dictum "physician heal thyself." In ancient civilizations, physicians were noted for their brilliant minds and far-reaching knowledge; they were society's thinkers, whose theories about health formed only a small part of an encompassing philosophy.

Our doctors are required only to graduate from a sanctioned medical school and to pass state boards. They are not expected to know anything about art, culture, and philosophy—let alone about the spirit. The idea that physicians heal themselves before healing others is no longer remotely entertained either by physicians or by those they presume to heal. In fact, if suicide rate, divorce rate, and drug and alcohol addiction rates can be taken as indicators, doctors are among the least healthy members of our society. A study of suicides committed between 1979 and 1988, conducted by the National Institute of Occupational Safety and Health, found that the odds of physicians committing suicide was 2.88 times greater than that of the general public, and among psychologists, it was 3.47 times greater.[33]

Prior to modern medicine, which I would date from the time of Louis Pasteur (circa 1850), medicine straddled the domains of both the physical and the metaphysical. In ancient societies, demons, magical actions and objects, the gods, or God, were believed to be primary sources of good or bad health. There was also, however, at all times, an accompanying strain of belief in purely material causes of disease and wellness. It is this strain, supported by the invention of new technologies, that we find triumphant in modern medicine.

Technology was and is the track that carries medical theory. I have no doubt that medicine became a study of the material person—not his mind or spirit—because instruments were invented that could measure the material world. I offer just two typical examples of the way medical materialism came to dominate medical theory: In the Middle Ages, Girolamo Fracastoro, a Veronese physician, believed that he proved Lucretius's atomic seed theory when he demonstrated that a person could contract an infection by coming in contact with a garment worn by an infected person.[34] Hundreds of years later, in Germany, Athanasius Kircher (1601–1680), using the compound microscope, actually saw "germs," thus confirming germs as the cause of disease. But neither Fracastoro nor Kircher would have found it possible to demonstrate—using infected materials, microscopes, or any other material object—the reason certain people who were exposed to infectious diseases, even the bubonic plague, did not contract the disease.

Similarly, Sanctorius's (1561–1636) invention of a chair scale allowed him to discover that his weight after a day of eating did not equal his original weight plus the weight of the food he had eaten, which led him to a primitive theory of metabolism.[35] But no scale is able to measure the inner malaise—the mental or spiritual disturbance—that could eventuate in metabolic disorders or obesity or emaciation.

Technology continues to drive medical history. We ask the questions we have the tools to answer, and the answers we arrive at allegorize the tools: the human body can be accessed by mechanical means; thus, the human being is a "machine."

Today's medical model did not evolve out of the free marketplace of ideas. It is a product of the practices of powerful physicians, of medical institutions, and of government policies.

At the time of the American Revolution, American medicine was a combination of folklore (the medicine of the people) and the "book medicine" or "high medicine" imported from European universities (the medicine of the specialist). Folk medicine, also called botanic medicine, combined the lore of the American Indians with remedies brought from the Old Country to produce a medicine that could be practiced by any layperson. America's first two medical schools, one in Philadelphia and the other in New York, obviously would teach high medicine, the medicine of the university-trained doctor.

High medicine was Hippocratic. It rested on the ancient Greek belief in the four humours (blood, phlegm, yellow bile, and black bile) that corresponded to the four elements of the universe (earth, air, fire, and water). Too much of one of the humours, it was believed, caused disease. Hippocratic medicine was "high" because it was too complicated to be performed by an ordinary person—it required a specialist to raise the temperature of the patient so much that it "cooked" the excess humour. The cooked humour would then be evacuated by bloodletting and bowel purging; by emetics, which induced vomiting; and by sudorifics, which induced sweating. These extreme measures became known as "heroic" medicine.

Heroic medicine often proved to be more lethal than the ailments it was supposed to cure. The most

famous doctor in America at the time of the
Revolutionary War was one Benjamin Rush—professor,
physician to the president, and disciple of William
Cullen (a Scottish physician). Cullen ascribed all illness
to capillary tension, and in some cases "heroically"
advocated removing as much as four-fifths of all the
blood in the body.

Rush, who also was a personal friend of the president and a ranking medical officer in the Revolutionary
Army, enjoyed social and political prominence that gave
him enormous power over the medical practices of the
day. He carried heroic medicine to the limits of its
destructiveness. When Philadelphia was struck with an
epidemic of yellow fever in 1793, Rush's recommended
treatment was massive bleeding combined with a purge
consisting of 15 grains of jalap and 10 grains of calomel
to be given every six hours. If the patient did not
improve, he was to be bled again and the dose of calomel
was to be increased to as much as 80 grains a day—a
lethal dose. Patients who survived this immediate assault
upon their bodies often succumbed more slowly to
calcification of the intestines—a condition, as autopsies
showed, widely suffered by soldiers in the Revolutionary
Army.

George Washington himself was a long-term victim
of his friend's "heroic" efforts. In small, continued
doses, calomel causes loose teeth and loss of hearing;
both were chronic complaints of Washington. In the end,
Washington died of what could have remained just a
cold. The day after the president came down with a cold
(Friday, December 13, 1799) his plantation foreman bled

him of 12 or 14 ounces, as instructed. The following day, two more copious bleedings were performed. Then he was dosed with calomel. After that, he was bled once again, this time of about a quart of blood. Later, he was given vapors of vinegar and water to inhale and another 10 grains of calomel, succeeded by repeated doses of tartar to induce vomiting. He died that night.[36]

We might scoff now at these barbaric methods, but they were the accepted medical practices of the day. Today's science is incontrovertible only until tomorrow's science controverts it; no book is more outdated than an old medical book. In the future, won't we regard currently accepted treatments as barbaric? In the treatment of some cancers, for example, after cutting patients, we poison them, then we bombard the affected area with radioactive rays that destroy whatever they touch.

There is no proof that the ascendancy of today's medical model was due to the intrinsic superiority of this model. We do have proof that free competition did not come into play, but that, instead, powerful societal forces installed and protected one school of thought. Medicine as taught by the established medical schools—later sanctioned by the American Medical Association (AMA), supported by the government, and rewarded by insurance companies—won out over the contenders.[37] Although during the past 15 or 20 years they have been gaining some resurgence, alternatives such as homeopathy, botanic medicine, faith healing, chiropractic, osteopathy, and naturopathy—which were thriving around the turn of the century—are now employed as adjuncts to conventional medicine by a small minority of the population. And almost nobody employs them as replacements for conventional medicine.

The medical saga of one group of people, the Mormons, serves as a revealing example of how one type of medicine came to monopolize the practice of medicine in America. In their early days, Mormons practiced a combination of botanic medicine (bolstered by prohibitions against tea, coffee, alcohol, and tobacco) and faith healing—calling upon Christ to enter the body of the sick person. When the Church of Jesus Christ of Latter-day Saints grew from a handful of struggling members to a sizable wealthy community, it built church hospitals where botanic medicine and faith healing were included in the treatment.

Today, Mormons constitute an even larger and wealthier community, yet Mormon hospitals have disappeared from the medical landscape—not because botanic medicine and faith healing didn't work, but because Mormon hospitals could not compete financially with hospitals that received money from the government. Government assistance came packaged with regulations that permitted only certain types of treatment—just as today Medicaid and Medicare reimburse only specific procedures approved by the American Medical Association. When the government extended funding to competing hospitals for buildings as well as administration, the competition became too great to withstand, and the last Mormon hospital shut down in 1974. Church leaders then, abandoning core Mormon beliefs about sickness and health, assured their followers that the use of "*the best medicine available*" does not indicate weakness in faith.[38] (Italics mine.)

I am not trying to promote either Mormon faith healing or botanic medicine. My point is that while organized medicine gives the illusion of choice, with its many doctors and many hospitals, it is as much a monopoly as we would have if Coca Cola, bottled under hundreds of different names, were the only beverage.

The medical monopoly was codified in 1910 by the Flexner Report.[39] Funded by the Carnegie Foundation for the Advancement of Teaching, the report endorsed standardized training and licensing and the accreditation of only certain schools. The influence of the AMA, the principal standard-bearer of Flexner principles, managed to drive out by law or stigma all practitioners who didn't meet Flexner qualifications. A new dichotomy was born: medicine and alternative medicine. Most people, then as now, could not afford alternative medicine, because neither the government nor private insurance companies help pay for it.

Medicine rests on a tradition of the superior being, one who possesses exclusive knowledge of the causes of things and whose powers accumulate in the tools of his trade—its charts and specialized argot, its mysterious nostrums. In ancient times, these tools were astrology and magical chants. Today, they are CAT scanners and

unpronounceable drugs. And the public is convinced
that the doctor, supported by an intimidating array of
technologies, knows best.

We can hardly blame doctors for this state of affairs.
The rock-bottom assumption of all medical school
education is that medicine has evolved from the muck of
primitive error to the present state of enlightenment.
Statements that might adjust this distorted judgment are
as rare as they are true. The 1983 graduates of Harvard
Medical School probably thought that Dean Burwell was
joking when he said, "Half of what we have taught you
is wrong. Unfortunately we do not know which half."[40]

And so, back to the routine checkup: It implies
that health is not normal and sickness is not aberrant.
It reminds us that we can become sick at any moment.
It tells us, in fact, that sickness may be in us at *this* very
moment, even though we feel fine. The routine checkup
enriches doctors by inculcating the patient's "sickness
mentality."

The routine checkup is justified because supposedly
it "catches" a minor disorder that if not caught might
become major. The myth promulgated by the medical
industry promises that the doctor can prevent your
dying. However, many authorities in the field of medicine itself claim that 80 percent of illnesses cure
themselves. If you are lucky enough not to have "early
detection," most disorders would simply disappear in
the course of the natural healing processes of the body.

But when a doctor detects a disorder at its incipient stage he or she medicates it. Now you are not a person but a patient; now you are worried; and now begins a second or third disorder—those side effects (whether you notice them or not) caused by *all* medication, bar none. Without early detection your mind would remain at peace, your immune system intact, and the disorder might well go away by itself.

Eighty percent of our ailments could heal themselves, yet we do not permit nature to take its healing course. Consider these facts:

1. One and a half billion visits to the doctor are made each year, and hospital admissions total 40 or 50 million!

2. Many thousands of hospital patients develop some kind of nosocomial infection—infection acquired during the hospital stay. In 1978, for example, one and a half million hospital patients were so afflicted[41]—and the number has grown, not decreased.

3. Thousands of patients receive the wrong treatment as a result of misdiagnosis.

4. Thousands develop new illnesses associated with the side effects of their medication, or surgery, or from unsuspected allergies.

5. Many patients are victims of mechanical equipment failures, especially in intensive care units.

When you add to all of this the hosts of miscellaneous small mistakes that occur, and when you also consider that 80 percent of illnesses simply go away without attention from a physician, you might reconsider the ramifications of the doctor visit.

In 1976, in his book *Limits to Medicine*, Ivan Illich wrote scathingly of iatrogenic disease—diseases caused by the physician: "The pain, dysfunction, disability, and anguish resulting from technical medical intervention now rival the morbidity due to traffic and industrial accidents and even war-related activities, and make the impact of medicine one of the most rapidly spreading epidemics of our time."[42] In 1987, Robert Peel extended the danger Illich spoke of to include periontogenic diseases. These are diseases caused by "things about" the patient, such as respirators and electrical hazards, that can result in casualties such as induced arrhythmias, burns, outright electrocutions, and infectious invasions.[43]

7

human machine/human statistic

In the sick room, ten cents' worth
of human understanding equals
ten dollars' worth of medical science.

—Martin. H. Fisher

Statistical tables that track the progress and mortality of cancer patients do not include me. Lolette Kuby, after appearing as a tubular carcinoma in the biopsy reports of Suburban General Hospital, dated January 26, 1982, becomes no doctor's patient and drops out of sight. She surfaces again in December 1989 as a lumpectomy performed by Doctor Lawrence Levy at Mount Sinai Hospital and then disappears again. No data anywhere say that, having refused all conventional treatment, 15 years later she is well, happy, and writing a book on the placebo effect that explains the phenomenon of her healing. She is not a stat, and having taken herself out of the medical loop, she has reclaimed her body from its former status as mechanism.

I am certainly not the first to observe that contemporary society reduces us to numbered objects—nowhere more harmfully than in our role as patient. The horrific procedures of heroic medicine have been left behind, but the perception of the human being as an object to be manipulated continues in full force. Almost everyone believes that something in the makeup of a human being could be called the psyche, and most people believe there is also a soul. Yet most of us also believe that illness originates and resides in matter—for example, in the colon, the kidney, the larynx, or the cerebral cortex.[44]

Whatever identities you hold in life—poet, artist, priest, plumber, homemaker—in the doctor's office you are reduced to flesh. You could be Mother Teresa, but in the reception room you join the other fidgeting or blank-faced or embarrassed or nervous or frightened bodies sitting in a row, usually long after the time of the scheduled appointments. (Downtime between patients cuts into profits.) Finally in the examining room, you disrobe, cover yourself with a minishift made of paper and, as instructed, lie down on a narrow table for another 15 or 20 minutes—this time without even a magazine. You never complain, of course, because a complaint would bring the reprimand that the doctor is busy with far more serious cases than yours. At last the doctor enters, with interrogations targeted specifically to the complaint:

What part is it that is racing, thumping, itching, or throbbing? you're asked. (Specialists, in particular, carry singleness of concern to the nth degree). The doctor then removes just that section of the paper shift that hides the malfunctioning part, as though your head bone were not connected to your hipbone, and neither was connected to anything that cannot be palpated.

After the diagnosis, you're fixed with tools that are cleaner than, but otherwise much the same as, the tools of a carpenter or an auto mechanic: wrenches, hammers, saws, pincers, pliers, and drills. Then you're given a prescription for chemicals to smear on or swallow, which Monsanto and Dupont produce in the same factories in which they manufacture bug killer and rust remover.

The destructiveness of all this goes far beyond any temporary psychic discomfort. A "victim mentality" and a mechanistic view of our own being begins in infancy. Doctors handle us as though we were material, so we learn to feel like material. Doctors seem not to care that they damage their own humanity in the process. Practitioner and patient mirror each other: If the patient is reduced to a mechanism, the doctor is a mechanic— and a mechanic is nothing without his tools. How different the relationship must have been when the doctor had to lay his ear to the patient's chest to hear the heart or lungs.

If we could detach our body parts and send them out to be fixed while we continued with our mental and spiritual life, mechanistic medicine would be a grand time-saver. Unfortunately, medicine treats our body as though, in fact, it were detached from our mind and soul. We are a "tumor," or "appendix," or "gall bladder." If one of these ailments sends us to the hospital, we're installed in a port where machines monitor our functions; nurses record the functions on a chart that hangs at the foot of the bed; and doctors arrive to peruse the chart, often without even a glance at the occupant of the bed. People have acquired, as Ivan Illich points out, "iatrogenic bodies. . . . They perceive themselves and their bodies as doctors describe them."[45]

As the scientific/technological approach to medicine rose, humanistic medicine fell. The epigraph quoted at the beginning of this chapter is laughably outdated. Ten dollars will not buy a crumb of medical science today, and human understanding—which one would think would be free as air—is as metered as a taxi ride. In today's medical schools, a course in human relations is considered avant garde. In 1983, it was necessary for Derek Bok, president of Harvard University, to seek the approval of the Board of Overseers to include "New Pathway" in the curriculum, a program designed to teach medical students something about the "emotional, psychological, and cultural substructure of human behavior."[46] "New Pathway," in other, less academic, words would teach future doctors how to humanize their behavior—what used to be called "bedside manner."

In 1986, *Psychology Today* published a study based on 800 tape-recorded pediatric visits to a hospital outpatient clinic. The study showed that the attention of doctors and medical staff focused almost exclusively on information gathering and on technology. Gestures of friendliness toward patients were absent even to the omission of everyday courtesies, including greetings and handshakes.[47]

Horror stories are told about surgery performed on the wrong part of the body or on the wrong person. Obviously these mistakes could not happen if the patient were a personality to the surgeon, rather than a shrouded anonymity with only the part of the anatomy exposed that the patient brought in to be repaired.

The small flurry of human-relations concerns that have found their way into Harvard and a minority of other medical schools might be encouraging if the underlying principle of bedside manners were recognized—that is, if it were recognized that the body and the mind of the patient comprise a single entity. But the Harvard course and those like it present compassion and understanding as accessories to treatment, a kind of decoration, rather than as an essential component of the treatment itself. If a doctor is not very compassionate or understanding, his problem is seen as a lack of communication skills or as a block in his emotions, not as a deficiency in his medical skills.

The recent effort to humanize doctors is spurred more by moral than medical concerns. It just isn't nice to make a patient feel like a helpless object. It isn't nice to patronize the patient or to take on the role of a supreme power. Sometimes it can even be dangerous. For example, it wasn't until a patient committed suicide that one doctor learned the value of empathy. Now he says, "I try to be as open-ended as possible when I talk to them. I've learned to tune in to what the patient is not telling me.

The more I pay attention to all aspects of the patient's life, the more I understand the person, the better I can tailor my approach to him."[48] Well and good, but one must wonder how doctors could ever have behaved differently.

Of course a doctor should shake your hand and know more of you than your diseased kidney! Of course the technology the doctor uses will be more effective if you are relaxed. It's almost beyond comprehension that these ideas should occur today as cutting-edge concepts.

Monetary considerations surely intrude on empathy; humane interactions cut into profits. "It might sound crude to compare a sick person to a retail customer," says one doctor, "but you don't need an MBA to figure out that the more patients you can see in the course of a day, the more revenue you can generate."[49] It takes far less time to write a prescription for a migraine headache than to sit down with the patient and explore what is troubling him. Moreover, even if it were proven that kindly interaction enhances the rate of cures, insurance companies and the government reimburse doctors by the number of patients they see, not by the number they cure. Unfortunately for all of us, the more people are sick, the more money is made.

Hospitals, clinics, and medical laboratories are businesses like any other business. And judging by the amount hospitals advertise, the competition to fill beds is far more fierce than the competition to fill machine-shop stalls.

If the number of beds exceeds the number of sick, it is tempting to encourage sickness. Because people do not go directly from their homes to hospitals, except in emergencies, we are constantly persuaded by pharmaceutical companies, government agencies, and doctors to visit the middleman—the doctors themselves. Insurance companies, of course, are *all* business: They promote the fear of illness in order to sell policies, but they deny the illness when the time comes to pick up the tab.

Machine functions can be measured by instruments and statistically tabulated. Individual humans cannot be so measured and so tabulated without disregarding the infinite number of variables that contribute to any human condition. Nonetheless, medical practices are based on statistics. Your demographic profile—your age, your gender, your race—rather than you as an individual, guides your doctor in the assessment and treatment of your illness. If you are a 50-year-old female, you are perceived differently than a 30-year-old man, no matter the actual condition of your body.

If that weren't bad enough, demographic profiles are established by a sick population. The validity of psychotherapy has been questioned because its theories stem from a disturbed group of people. The entire field of medicine can be challenged on the same basis. The many people who do not seek medical attention at all, and those who visit alternative medicine practitioners exclusively, do not exist in medical statistical tables. Whether they are healthier or less healthy, live longer or die earlier than the rest of the population, the medical industry does not know and perhaps is afraid to find out.

Their fear is understandable: The scant research that

has been done in this area suggests that people who do not go to doctors perhaps are healthier than those that do. But are they naturally healthier and *therefore* do not go to doctors? Or, are they healthier *because* they do not go to doctors? A Utah study may suggest the latter. Taking a random group of Mormons, the study found a significantly lower incidence of cancer and heart disease than in the general population. Could that lower rate have anything to do with the fact that many Mormons still practice faith healing and herbal healing in their own homes?[50]

The best-known group that does not enter medical statistics is Christian Science. Its constituents don't go to doctors and don't participate in medical research, so there is no way of knowing who among them is sick or who has been healed without medical attention. But we do know that evidence of nonmedical healing crams Christian Science literature, and Christian Science graveyards are not cluttered with bodies of those who have died young.[51]

In today's medicine, statistics color perception, structure expectation, and dictate treatment. You are expected to have elevated blood pressure at a certain age, or poor eyesight, or more porous bones, or trembling hands—only because correlations have been found between these conditions and given ages. When you reach these ages, the maladies associated with them are deemed to be *normal* for you.

That disease is normal is an article of faith, a dogma, for most doctors. A very few doctors have shifted to a different perception of human health, some even abandoning the practice of medicine altogether. (See chapter 17, "Breakthrough Medicine.") But most of the medical industry believes that health is predicated upon disease: Underneath health lies illness, like a trap door.

How does all of this relate to the placebo effect?

Orthodox medicine is centered on ideas that accentuate the mechanical functioning of the human being. Contrary ideas that emerge from the fields of psychology and sociology make little dent in the medical model, and ideas that come from fields of metaphysics make no dent at all. Orthodox medicine simply contains no *conceptual* base for fundamentally dealing with the following reality: A sugar pill can change symptoms; a sugar pill can alter organic conditions.

A few doctors are so skeptical of the role the mind plays in health that they deny that such a thing as a placebo effect exists. To them it proves nothing more than that the disease that disappeared must have never really existed. Most doctors, however, do admit the reality of that "nuisance" phenomenon, but they look away from its mind-boggling implications. Understandably, doctors feel greatly threatened; for, if the placebo effect is both ubiquitous and powerful, where does that leave the medical model most doctors observe?

Conventional medicine claims that because its approaches are based on science, its findings are both *reliable* and *provable*, while metaphysical areas like faith healing, psi phenomena, and placebo effects, are neither. But conventional medicine has come up with its own definition of "reliable" and "provable," and it imposes higher standards of reliability and provability on any deviating practice. For example, faith healers are expected to be unconditionally reliable: They are expected to cure anyone of anything at the exact moment under investigation. If the faith healer is unable to do this in a laboratory situation, it is taken as evidence of the fraudulence of the healer or of faith healing in general.

Likewise, in laboratory experiments, telepaths are expected to read the mind of a particular person at a particular moment of time. A telepath who fails may be dubbed a charlatan, and the whole area of mind reading may be regarded as hokum. But a doctor's misdiagnoses are regarded as reasonable and expected occasional errors. And if a particular patient fails to benefit from a certain treatment, it is regarded as the patient's biological individuality.

Because they often cannot be replicated at will, thousands of recorded cases of faith healing do not penetrate the obstinate materialism of biomedical thinking. Yet thousands of recorded medical misdiagnoses and hundreds of thousands of treatments that do patients minimal good fail to shake that thinking.

Aside from intentional omission, there is a plausible reason for the paucity of medical research into faith healing or into the spontaneous disappearance of disease, a reason that points to a flaw inherent in the scientific method—that is, the necessity of replication to test the validity of the finding. If a cancer has vanished, what does one investigate? Medicine can measure the patient's blood, urine, and the like, before and after—but these are physiological details, not explanations for the disappearance. The destruction of human tissue by radiation can be replicated in the laboratory. But if that same tissue has been regenerated by faith healing, there is no way to repeat the regeneration.

The other side of this unmanageable coin is the fact that science can't tell who is "really" sick. Laboratory tests of a healthy person can show a whole host of factors that show up also in sick people. In other words, a healthy person might harbor in his or her body an array of disease-related organisms, abnormal tissue, and malfunctioning organs, yet feel and act healthy. For example, postmortem examinations of people who died in automobile accidents have revealed widespread incidence of cancer cells, yet these people had displayed no symptoms of cancer. "What looks like cancer under the microscope does not always act like cancer in the living body." The incidence of cancer of the thyroid, prostate, and uterus, for instance, discovered post-mortem is actually greater than its apparent prevalence in life.[52]

The human being perceived as machine and the failure to take seriously the placebo effect go hand in glove. The placebo effect is an effect with no external cause—it is a function of faith. And while faith may be cultivated or stimulated by external triggers (see chapter 19), these triggers are infinite in quantity. Biomedicine is equipped to deal only with measurable material causes in material entities. As the old adage says, "If your only tool is a hammer, you will see all problems as nails."

8

the myriad modes of alternative medicine

On the subject of singing,
the frog school and the lark school disagree.

—*Chinese proverb*

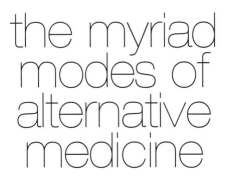

I refused conventional cancer treatment, but a couple of weeks after the diagnosis I did visit one MD. He practiced alternative medicine in association with a pediatrician who defected from his status position at the Cleveland Clinic after he became convinced of the destructiveness of conventional medical treatment. My doctor viewed cancer as an imbalance in the body's chemistry. He treated it with vitamin and mineral supplements and diet. As I understand it, the aim was to heighten immune function, rid the body of toxins, and decrease cell oxidation. These corrections were to enable the body to rid itself of the cancer.

On the first of my two visits, I was startled to see one room filled with people who were sitting in lounge chairs and were hooked up for hours to some sort of intravenous equipment—but the receptionist assured me that I wouldn't have to go through this. These were chelation patients, most likely arthritis sufferers, who were having their bodies flushed of accumulations of heavy metals.

My entire treatment consisted of an intake interview, a thermography—which shows diseased tissue as hot spots (mine was cool)—a wide spectrum of laboratory tests, including a hair analysis, and an exit interview. The doctor, seeming far more concerned with the chemical imbalance indicated by my complaint that I was always hungry than with the cancer, painstakingly explained the relationship between oxidation and disease and prescribed a special diet and supplements. Nevertheless, the entire process, though far less traumatic than a visit to the Cleveland Clinic, was impersonal and could have been conducted by a laboratory robot and a television MD. The doctor did not touch me, nor inquire into the state of my mind or emotions.

Vitamin supplements had been part of my diet most of my adult life and still are.[53] The newly prescribed supplements eliminated calcium and introduced a high dose of pantothenic acid, but otherwise contained much of what I had already been taking—but in a considerably more costly compound formulated by the doctor. I would need to return in a couple of months to replenish the supply; no other appointment was scheduled.

I am not denigrating this doctor's practice. These and other alternative measures are more effective, less expensive, and far less damaging than conventional procedures. However, I did not return a third time, partly because Blue Cross refused to cover vitamin therapy, but mostly because with each passing day I was gaining the courage of my conviction that biomedicine, even more gentle biomedicine, is not the source of healing.

A trickle of doctors have left the practice of conventional medicine and have taken up some type of alternative medicine. A heavier trickle, probably more than would care to admit, have incorporated alternative therapies into orthodox practices. Of a random sampling of 250 doctors, about half confessed to using unconventional methods, but didn't want to be identified for fear their peers would ridicule them.[54]

Some medical schools, among them Harvard and Georgetown, have introduced guided imagery, acupuncture, biofeedback training, and a few other alternative medicine therapies, even Qi Gong, into their curriculum. Perhaps they are influenced by the rising income potential of alternative medicine—estimated in 1999 by the National Institutes of Health (NIH), Office of Alternative Medicine (OAM), to be $13 billion a year.

Conventional medicine faces a dilemma that only the most open-minded doctors are willing to face. This dilemma shows up clearly in the controversy about Norman Cousins. In his book *Anatomy of an Illness*, Cousins proclaims that he cured himself of ankylosing spondylitis (a degenerative disease of the connective tissue) by adopting a healthy mental attitude, by laughing a lot, and by taking extremely high doses of vitamin C. I'm certain that Cousins's far-out story would have been utterly disregarded had he not been a famous man. Yet despite his prominence, his claims were denigrated by many doctors, who argued that Cousins must have misrepresented the nature and the severity of his illness, because ascorbic acid, risibility, and optimism could in no way affect collagen disorder.

Cases analogous to Cousins's probably occur by the thousand, but remain unknown. Only his fame and access to publishers and the media allowed his experience to be publicized. Perhaps his case influenced some doctors to conform less rigidly to medical orthodoxy and encouraged some people to take greater responsibility for their own health. One consequence of his story was the start of a new alternative medicine: laughter therapy. Now, people with cancer assemble to laugh together, sometimes for hours and sometimes for days—and they swear that it helps them.

Practically any therapy that occupies little or no place within the canon of orthodox medicine is gathered under the rubric "alternative medicine," which encompasses a huge grab bag of philosophies and techniques widely different from one another. Yoga, Creative visualization, the Alexander Technique, crystal therapy, Reiki, therapeutic touch, homeopathy, Transcendental

Meditation™, The Feldenkrais Method®, hands-on
therapy, music and sound therapy, color therapy, chakra
adjustment, aura adjustment, acupressure, chiropractic,
vibration and magnet therapy, massotherapy, herbal
therapy, macrobiotics, juice fasting and other cleansing
therapies, Pritikin® and other diet therapies, shiatsu,
CranioSacral manipulation, Electroacuscope, Ayurveda,
and many more are all regarded as alternatives to conventional medicine.

Can all of these therapies—so diverse, so utterly
different from one another (some of them so downright
odd)—really be effective? Of course they can: If the
patient believes in their efficacy, they are placebos, and
the healing that follows their use is a placebo effect, an
effect whose cause is really *internal* although an outward
agent is given the credit.

Alternative therapies can be classified according to
their primary focus—the body, the mind, or the spirit.
Some manipulate or adjust limbs and organs; some
emphasize a return to nature using herbal medication,
vegan diet, or other means of reconnecting with Mother
Earth; some employ a peculiar assortment of instruments
like crystals, which are believed to have supernatural
attributes that can affect mind or body; and some concentrate on spiritual or quasi-religious ritual activities.
Unlike modern medicine, which seems to change daily—
each "cure" nipping at the heels of a previous cure,
which only yesterday was touted as the cure—alternative
therapies have antecedents in ancient religions, philosophies, and folklores.

The distinction I find most critical in evaluating

alternative therapies is that some require the intervention of an external agent—whether person or object—and others do not. The latter group would include autosuggestion, TM and other meditation practices, biofeedback training, and Reiki. A guru or highly experienced person may be engaged in the training process, but at some point the individual learns to practice the technique on himself or herself to accomplish self-healing.

Many alternative medicine therapies are based on the idea that the body has points—called chakras, meridians, or plexes—that can be manipulated or adjusted to control mental and physical health. These target points are not recognized in the anatomy charts of conventional medicines, but are chronicled in the literature of remarkably far-flung cultures and across eons of time. In ancient Greece, for example, certain occultists believed that the spine (corresponding to the vertebrae of the god Osiris), marked the stations of a mystical ladder. An order of Orthodox monks in today's Greece continues the tradition, locating six plexus points—forehead, throat, heart, solar plexus (below the rib cage), sex organs, and "tail" (the bottom of the spine). Hindus identify this tail plexus—the perineum-sacroiliac area—as the *kundalini,* the seat of sexual passions and prowess, which can be trained to "rise" to become mental/spiritual energy. The Latin word for this area, *sacrum,* may be the historical root of the word "sacred."[55] From ancient times to the present, these points have been adjusted by needles or by hands or through meditation to transmit life energy, promote clear thinking, reduce stress, and generally to give a sense of well-being and balance.

Other therapies adjust points or energies that never did and never will appear in anatomical diagrams because they are not part of the physical body at all, but are emanations from the body. Such is the "crown chakra" or *sahasrara*, recognized by Hindus and Buddhists. It is located just above the head, where the physical and transcendent worlds meet. In Christianity, this spot is exactly the place of the halo as depicted in pictures of Jesus, Mary, and the Saints.

During a treatment of one of these disembodied points, the therapist's hands will flutter around the body, never touching it, to massage and move and adjust what seems to be only air. This "air," however, is an etheric or psychomagnetic field, which occultists always have claimed exists—a claim that in modern times seems to be confirmed in Kirlian photography. Kirlian photography captures on film an image, not visible to the naked eye, that surrounds the body and changes in color and intensity depending on the subject's mood and physical condition.

At the other extreme are alternative medicine therapies that rely on the properties of objects and instruments, including magnets, copper bracelets, needles, and electrical vibrators. But unlike the technological hardware of conventional medicine—tools analogous to hammers and chisels—alternative medicine devices are said to derive their power from cosmic forces of one kind or another. For example, magnets plug into the gravitational pulls of earth, moon, stars, and planets. The electroscope utilizes the constant vibrational state of atomic and subatomic particles. And crystals, the most widely known of alternative medicine objects, possess a kind of supernatural energy, depending on their size, clarity, color, and geological type; the energy transfers to those who wear them, carry them, place them in their environments, or meditate upon them.

One of the newest alternative therapies, color therapy, uses color to modify moods and emotions. Like yoga or meditation, it is capable of quieting the mind and relaxing the body. Our language reflects our awareness that color and emotions are intimately tied: When we are angry, we "see red"; when sad, we "feel blue"; when frightened, we behave like a "yellow coward." Color therapy uses lights, cloths, and ambient color to make the patient feel tranquil and happy. Studies have proven that children calm down in a pale blue room and act up in a room decorated in bright reds and greens.

One of the oldest therapies, probably predating Pythagoras's idea of the harmony of the spheres, uses musical sounds to calm the individual and heighten spiritual awareness. Buddhist temple bells; bowls made of crystal; the human voice singing, speaking, or chanting—virtually any object with harmonic capability—can promote health and healing. The Buddhist chant "Om Mani Padme Hum" supposedly resonates with the universe. Conversely, as we all know, a chalk grating across a blackboard can set our teeth on edge. We can only speculate about the effect sound pollution in a modern industrial city has on health.

Poetry therapy, drama therapy, and art therapy— once considered ridiculous by orthodox psychologists— have become acceptable as research has proven their value in healing the body as well as the mind. And music not only soothes the savage beast, but strains of Mozart or Brahms have been shown to make plants grow.

Until less than a hundred years ago, alternative medicine was mainstream medicine. Folklore and herbal remedies competed successfully with medical school doctors. If you were sick, you were just as likely to be treated by a "botanic" doctor as by a "book-learned" doctor. The most famous botanic medicine was Thomsonianism, named after its founder, Samuel Thomson, a kind of one-man pharmacopoeia. As a young boy, Thompson had chewed on lobelia leaves, a powerful emetic, and learned a lesson about nature's potency he never forgot. In adulthood, he investigated the properties of every plant he came across. Sometimes he applied the ancient doctrine of signatures: the belief that objects in nature resemble the part of the body they're to be used to remedy—the forked mandrake root, for instance, for female genital problems. Thompson bottled his nostrums and distributed them through a network that resembles contemporary franchises.[56] Today, Thompson would be called a snake oil salesman, but in the late years of the nineteenth century, his patented medicines benefited many a sick person.

The practices of premodern medicine almost always had metaphysical import. Many of today's alternative medicines revive these metaphysical foundations. Sound therapy, for example, is backed up by a far-reaching spiritual tradition: Sound played so great a part in the mysteries of Eleusis that a man with a defective voice was not permitted to participate. In eleventh-century

England, a choir admitted into the sickroom could bring a cure by intoning the daily offices. In India, the dreaded class of seers known as the *Knaphata* or "ear-torn" yogis, to this day regard the ear as mystical: The blood that results from perforating the cartilage during initiation ceremonies is believed to stream from a hidden holy channel and is used to anoint the head. In the Bible, music could whip a Hebrew prophet into a frenzy of passionate excitement or, in the mouth of David, could cool the choler of a raging king.

Every herb that grows on earth—plus the bark, seed, root, or leaf of every tree, plus soil and stones—all probably have been used at some time in some society to cure someone of something. Common today are chamomile for relaxation, ginger for nausea, ginseng root for sexual potency, cloves for toothache, and St. John's Wort for depression. Folklore contains prescriptions far more exotic than these: In America, rainwater collected from hollow beech trees cured scurf and scabies, and beech-bark tea cured rheumatism; in Russia, a concoction made of lilac leaves forestalled aging; and in Greece, walking barefoot on freshly plowed earth alleviated mental disturbances.

Relatively few alternative practices have invaded conventional medicine. Among those that have, diet is the most common. Doctors do not leave their fields of study easily—they leave when in good conscience they cannot continue practices that do more harm than good.

Three physicians explain why they switched from the drugs and invasive procedures of conventional medicine to dietary medicine: "Much of the stuff that we got in medical school was in some way influenced by the pharmaceutical industry," says one. "I began to talk to alternative health practitioners and found they had good results, sometimes even better than what medical doctors were getting. We had been kind of hoodwinked in school. We were told that anybody who wasn't an MD was a quack."[57]

The second, who was a young cardiologist in 1980, realized "that no one was getting healed of cardiovascular disease. . . . I saw what Nathan Pritikin was accomplishing using diet and exercise." After this physician converted his practice to diet therapy, 90 percent of his heart patients went off their medication.[58]

The third, an anesthesiologist, experienced a "dramatic epiphany." He kept seeing fat people on the operating table, being operated on by fat surgeons "reaming out these big long yellow sausages of fatty material from the man's arteries." He wondered "if eating animal products is necessary at all," and eliminated all of them from his own diet. Deciding that he wanted to keep people off the operating table, he ended up in a small practice in Florida, where he installed a kitchen in his office and brought in a vegetarian cook to teach patients how to eat.[59]

The standard objection of conventional doctors to alternative medicine is that at best it endangers the patient by delaying his visit to a "real" doctor, and at worst it kills him. Considering that it is often those whom conventional treatment has failed—the very sickest segment of the sick population—who arrive at the doorstep of nonestablishment practitioners, the wonder is how many improve and live.

I have very ambivalent feelings about conventional medicine's adoption of any alternative medical practice. On one hand, I am happy to see traumatizing techniques accompanied by more moderate ones. On the other hand, while the growing new field of alternative medicine (identified by the labels "complementary" or "integrative" and led by such doctors as Andrew Weil) is liberalizing conventional medicine and pointing in the right direction toward true alternatives, it may actually impede more sweeping changes. Integrative medicine seems to be analogous to a meat eater who sits down to a big steak and says that by adding a helping of spinach he is integrating vegetarianism into his diet. The medical monolith can swallow and digest alternatives *without altering its basic paradigm*. Assimilation might well weaken rather than strengthen the possibility that alternative medicine can steer us toward a new way of thinking about health—a way far beyond its own procedures.

My greatest hope for the benefits of alternative medicine is that people who change their therapy may be ready to change their mind. My greatest disappointment is with those therapies that utilize external objects and external agents to produce physical changes. The agent may be an acupuncturist, the object may be a copper bracelet worn on an arthritic arm, but these are as "external" as surgeons and drugs.

When Dr. Richard M. Chin, an MD who uses
Eastern medical alternatives, explains the principles
behind Qi—balancing the opposing forces of yin and
yang—he doesn't refer to mind, emotions, or spirit, but
to blood vessels and organs. For example, he works on
energy blockages in the lung that may "upset the overall
balance of the body's entire energy system [and be] experienced as coughing, asthma, allergies, skin problems,
bronchitis, and fatigue."[60] Within the framework of
self-healing and the placebo effect, I see little difference
between the fundamental view of Dr. Chin and that of
typical Western doctors. Both correlate sickness with the
physical body and attempt healing by working directly
upon the body in one way or another.

Interestingly, Dr. Chin does make two observations
that, if he took seriously, might recast his own view of
medicine. He says, "Westerners strongly associate needles
with pain, instead of with relief from it." With this statement, Chin admits that pain is culturally determined
(e.g., in some cultures, cutting the hair is experienced as
painful), yet he doesn't seem to be aware that what he
has said implies that both pain and relief from pain
reside in the mind, not in the needle. He also says,
"There are some Westerners who discount the success
of acupuncture as being a kind of 'placebo' effect, that is,
results are realized *only because the patient believes it will
cure them.*"[61] (Italics mine.) So, despite his important
work in alternative medicine, like other doctors, his
desire to protect his particular specialty obscures the significance of placebo effects—cures that are accomplished
by belief alone.

Nevertheless, if I were forced to choose, I would choose alternative over conventional medicine as more nearly fulfilling Hippocrates's commandment: "First, do no harm." It is less invasive, has fewer side effects, costs less, causes less pain, and, most important, gives patients greater autonomy. Often it induces a state of relaxation and trustfulness, two conditions that do in fact promote healing. The patient is less involved in a battle with his own body or with malign influences such as bacteria. Conventional medicine declares war on the body; alternative medicine enlists the body's assistance.[62]

With so many alternative treatments to choose from, a person can go crazy trying to find the "right" one. To the list already mentioned can be added colonic flushes, rebirthing, past-life recovery, and drumming. I am certainly not acquainted with all of the choices, but my essential point is this: Anything can stimulate healing if you believe in it. If you believe that you will be healed when a butterfly lands on your nose, then you will be healed by a rhino-lepidoptera.[63] If you fully believe that you will die if bats invade your house, you will die; indeed, many people who had faith in the Bat Theory of Death, did die.

What can we call these effects? Health via butterfly? Demise via bat? Whatever we call them, they are placebo effects. They operate exactly as placebos operate in conventional medicine.

9

the power of the mind

O, the mind, mind has mountains, cliffs of fall
Frightful, sheer, no-man fathomed . . .
—G.M. Hopkins

I continued to feel a lump in my breast for eight
years, yet I knew at the deepest level of my being that
the cancer was cured. Whatever that lump was, it posed
no danger to my health and life. How had I become
cured? So many answers were offered from so many
quarters, but none jibed with my new understanding of
life. My religious friends believed that Jesus or God
had intervened with nature—in other words, a miracle
had occurred. My spiritual but nontheistic friends
thought some kind of cosmic energy had entered me. My
"scientific" friends implored me to have a mastectomy

and chemotherapy, and when I did neither, they waited for me to sicken and die. My continued health persuaded them that the diagnosis must have been mistaken, or that my own fear verbally elevated a benign tumor to the terrible status of cancer: "But did you actually have a biopsy?" "Yes." "By a genuine accredited laboratory?" "Yes. Yes."

Despite the skepticism and suspicion I encountered, I felt it was my duty to pass along what I had learned. But not having done so during these past few years, the feeling of obligation escalated to an intensity that could only be described as continuous guilt. I had been given a mission. I was not permitted to withhold from others what I knew. What those others would do with the message I could not control.

Continued good health is a door few know how to unlock. In this book I provide as many keys as I can think of to prove that there is only one source of health, one source of disease, and one source of healing: It is your *mind*, in the largest sense of that word—a composite of your beliefs about the very nature of reality and the nature of your own being. The healing power of the mind is not a miracle or a mystery, no more a mystery than that the eye can see, no more a miracle than mind itself. When the great skeptic Voltaire was asked whether he believed in reincarnation, he answered that he found it no more incredible that he should live many times than that he should live once. I apply his logic to health: It is no more incredible that you can heal a cancer than that you can heal a hangnail.

Every minute of our lives we are immersed in proofs of the mind's power: The placebo effect is only one of those proofs. Three others—the Hawthorne effect, self-fulfilling prophecy, and accident-proneness—in my opinion, are among the most important insights of modern psychology, but, as with the placebo effect, the magnitude of the implications of these phenomena has not been followed to a logical conclusion.

The Hawthorne effect is a phenomenon in which the control group shows as much improvement as the experimental group. The effect is named after the Western Electric Company's Hawthorne plant where an investigation on productivity yielded an unexpected outcome. The investigation was designed to measure the output of factory workers when brighter lighting was installed. Productivity did increase. But unexpectedly, the output of the control group, which worked under the old, dimmer lights, also increased. Both groups had been told they were participating in an experiment. The researchers concluded that not the lighting, but the workers' awareness of their role in an experiment made them work more efficiently. In other words, a thought in the mind was as effective as brighter lights. To test this serendipitous result, three groups were formed. The third worked under the old lighting but were not told they were being observed. Output of this third group remained at the old, lower level.

Of course the Hawthorne effect isn't a new capability of the human mind, but rather a new label that identifies the mind's inherent power. Likewise with self-fulfilling prophecy. Psychology's identification of self-fulfilling prophecy is enormously important, not only because it dethrones oracles, magicians, and configurations of the stars, but also because it sets individuals in their rightful place as the authors of their own fate. The prophet Samuel prophesied that the peasant Saul would become king of Israel. The oracle at Thebes prophesied Oedipus's fratricide and incest. That both came to pass was believed to fulfill the intention of the gods. But the concept of self-fulfilling prophecy explains the phenomena: The events came to pass because Saul and Oedipus *believed* the prophecies, and consequently—consciously or unconsciously—acted in such a way as to bring them about.

Self-fulfilling prophecy says that external forces do not determine the course of our lives, but rather it is our self-perception that structures what happens to us. As every psychologist knows, if you feel you are too stupid, inept, and unattractive to keep a job or find a girl, you lose the job and don't find the girl. If you feel that you are desirable and competent, the job and the girl more likely will be yours.

The concept of accident-proneness is similarly linked to the power of mind. As the label suggests, the mishaps of accident-prone people are not accidental. The accident-prone are *inclined* to put their body at risk. As the *Dictionary of Behavioral Science* defines it, these people act out and discharge unconscious impulses through accidents. They trip on the sidewalk, fall down the stairs, and get hit by flying objects. Their car brakes lock, their sharp knives slip, the stepladder rung gives way. Can the victims of such misadventures be blamed? Weren't they innocently standing under the scaffolding when the construction worker dropped the hammer? For me, it is easier to believe in demon possession than to believe these mishaps occur completely by chance.

Nor is it completely by chance that accidents do not happen. If the mind plays a role in the cause of accidents, you would also expect it to play a role in the avoidance of accidents—and it does. Some people have never suffered a broken bone or a sprained ankle. Some have escaped uninjured from catastrophes. These individuals seem to be surrounded by a protective shield—an accident unlikelihood or accident "a-susceptibility" that protects them from harm, yet they take no greater precautions and are no more safety-conscious than the rest of us. For example, in *The Road Less Traveled*, M. Scott Peck tells about an automobile accident from which the driver emerged unscathed out of a car that was crushed almost flat.

I believe that even a single accident reveals that the person's state of mind was accident-prone—if only for a moment—when the accident occurred. I have been both accident-prone and accident-resistant. I was accident-prone the day I jumped off a bed only two feet high and shaved my Achilles' heel on the metal bed frame. I was accident-prone the day I landed spread-eagled on the tennis court. And, I was accident-prone the day I slammed a door on my own finger. In the first instance, I was greatly agitated; in the second, highly self-conscious; and in the third, exceedingly angry. In all three instances, my mind was in one place and my body in another. By not keeping body and soul together, so to speak, I put my body in harm's way.

I was accident-resistant the day my family was dining at a glass-walled restaurant on the shores of Lake Erie when a tornado spun across the lake. Seconds before it struck, I intuited that the picture windows were going to blow, and within seconds herded my family into the safety of the restaurant kitchen. Others followed our lead. The accident-prone just sat there and were injured by flying glass. Even they, I think, came to their senses before the piano was hurtled around the room.

The Hawthorne effect, self-fulfilling prophecy, and accident-proneness are recognized and verified conditions of mind over matter. But what is rarely acknowledged is the probability that our minds control the events of our lives at all times and in every situation.

We have all heard of people who lift a weight far beyond the capacity of their musculature in order to save someone they love. What is it that infuses their limbs with this sudden puissance? Adrenaline, of course; but wasn't it a state of mind that sent the adrenaline surging? And how about the inebriated person who sobers up the instant police approach? And consider the fatigued person who runs like a track star when danger chases. And haven't we all joked about how much better we feel as soon as we're sitting in the doctor's office? One emergency room physician observes that symptoms seem to abate as soon as the sufferer has *made up his or her mind* to seek medical care.

Stress, which lately and rightfully has been implicated in almost every disease, is also a state of mind: There are no stressful situations, only stressed-out people. The same situation can enervate one person and invigorate another. One researcher points out that "the way in which the stress is dealt with—indeed, perceived—may deflect serious impact."[64] The emphasis, he says, should be put not so much on the stressors as on "the cognitive and coping processes mediating the reaction." It isn't the divorce, the transfer to another city, the job layoff, or the illness that causes the stress—it is the way you assess these events.

Healthy, vigorous octogenarians exemplify positive self-fulfilling prophecy. We constantly try to attribute happy longevity to physical lifestyle. We ask octogenarians what they ingest and imbibe. Do they smoke? Do they exercise? Their answers, however, point to their minds.[65]

Claude Pepper, who served in public office, including both houses of Congress, for five decades, said, "I'm as full of ideas about what to do in the future as a dog has fleas. . . . The Lord blessed me with a good temperament. That is, optimism. I don't think about what might happen, that I could step out my door and be run over by a bus. I think about what can be done today. I think about doing a good job in the here and now. So, psychologically, growing old doesn't affect me."

The painter Raphael Soyer said, "I face new challenges every day. I want to do larger, more complex compositions that will test my new skills and will be difficult to fulfill. Every painting I do is just as if I've never painted before."

Meridel LeSueur, a writer, said, "I don't admit age. I

call it ripening. . . . Ripening has distinct advantages for women—they have a chance to regain their full identity as a person. I'm just beginning to face a big challenge in my work—a new style, a more poetic vision, better images."

And Max Lerner said, "I work toward the affirmatives—love, work and the linkages between them. I used to think you never did anything for the first time as an old person, but only for the last time. It isn't true. I'm doing many things for the first time."

⁓

We need the term "illness-prone," or "self-fulfilling illnesses," to accurately indicate the true cause of disease. The term "psychosomatic illness" might do if it did not connote *all* in the mind instead of *originating* in the mind. The list of illnesses that even the medical industry associates with mental states becomes longer all the time: ulcers, colitis, anorexia, bulimia, and, lately, heart trouble and even cancer. If mind plays a role in those illnesses, why not in arthritis, and why not in the common cold? All illness is psychosomatic—it begins in the psyche. This is not a new idea: For example, almost two hundred years ago, the German mathematician August Möbius referred to goiter as "crystallized fear." And haven't most of us proven in our own experience that what we fear is more likely to happen? "Beliefs and expectations sicken and kill," acknowledges one doctor."[66]

Marx, Freud, and Einstein tower over twentieth century thought, no one more than Freud with his identification and analysis of the unconscious. But Freud's path was not uncharted; a hundred years earlier, the Austrian physician Franz Mesmer discovered the subconscious mind.

Initially, Mesmer found that through the use of magnets he could modify his patients' bodily functions. Later, he found that words alone—spoken very loudly, shouted at the patient—worked as well as magnets. Still later, he found that words alone—softly spoken and perhaps accompanied by something like a swinging pendulum—could induce a trance state; and during the trance, the patient could be instructed to alter bodily functions. Mesmer, in other words, made a threefold discovery: He could induce hypnotic trance, he could access the subconscious mind during the trance, and he could use the subconscious mind to alter physiological processes.[67]

In the years between Mesmer and Freud, one of Mesmer's students taught the art of hypnotism to Phineas Parkhurst-Quimby, an uneducated New England clockmaker. Quimby became an extraordinary hypnotist. At first, he used the theatrical devices of mirrors, pendulums, and stock phrases in vaudeville-type shows that people paid to attend. The profound import of the subject's suggestibility and the trance state didn't dawn on him until much later. When it did, he began to use hypnotism to heal.

Quimby's further enlightenment followed a life-threatening horse-and-buggy ride: Frightened by something, the horse pulling Quimby's carriage broke into a wild, uncontrollable careening run that required all of Quimby's strength and presence of mind to bring to a halt. Before this incident he had long suffered from severe back pains, which nothing could alleviate. Somehow, during the runaway his back was completely healed.

Quimby was not one to disregard this "miracle," or to see in it the hand of God—he was not a religious man in the usual sense of the word. He hypothesized that his back problem had originated in his mind and then was transferred to his body. Once the disorder was dislodged from his mind, as it had been during his extreme fright, it vanished from his body. From that day on, Quimby understood the principle behind hypnotic healing. His treatments were now conscious attempts, using hypnotism and every other technique he could think of, to change his patients' states of mind.

To Quimby, the correlation of body and mind was not a hypothesis. It was a law—what Quimby called a "science." The sick came from all over New England to partake of Quimby's science. Mary Baker Eddy, the founder of Christian Science, was one of the people who came for his help. She arrived from Boston to be healed of debilitating back problems and remained after her cure to be Quimby's student. In turn, she taught or influenced the leading figures of the New Thought movement, the spiritual/religious movement that evolved during the nineteenth century.

In one of the curiosities of modern history, at the
same time as medical science began to dominate the
general consciousness with its dogma of matter over
mind, New Thought expounded the power of mind over
matter. My own experience and my investigation into the
placebo effect leaves me no room for doubt that Quimby
was right—belief in illness is a cultural and personal
mystification; we literally hypnotize ourselves into a state
that alters bodily functions. As long as we remain in this
trance of illness, our bodies will continue to act out the
patterns of our thoughts.

Conversely, people can cultivate a state of mind that
manifests health and well-being, and it is this possibility
that is promulgated by all the gurus of the self-help
movement—from Norman Vincent Peale 50 years ago
to today's Wayne Dyer and Marianne Williamson. New
Thought groups, as well as some traditional religious
groups, use affirmations and creative visualization to
groove into the mind new and desirable ideas that are
expected to "produce after their kind." Affirmations are
verbal assertions that a desired state of being is already
in existence. Creative visualization is the immediate
"seeing" of a certain condition or event.

To most of us, the power of our mind and beliefs
to govern our health seems implausible, even though we
see that power proven continually in areas other than
health. We see the state of mind of a nation erupt into
the international violence called "war." We see the state

of mind of a community explode into race riots. Clearly, states of mind in the body politic translate into events. Clearly, the bullet in the victim existed first in the mind of the killer. Yet we can't believe that illness in our personal body existed first in our mind. Our consciousness is filled with illness and disease, yet we fail to—even refuse to—connect this with the illness and disease that show up in our body.

To some extent, psychotherapy, by definition, holds the mind responsible for the individual's state of being. Psychologists and psychiatrists—even those who seek the primary cause of illness in biology and external trauma—attempt to rid the psyche of habitual "wrong thinking" and to replace it with the "right thinking" that would allow the individual to change his or her life. Among the various schools of psychology, cognitive therapy, Logotherapy, Rational Emotive Therapy, and Gestalt therapy in particular recognize that health spreads from an internal state to an external state: What you say in your mind, your "self-talk," molds your experience.

We live not with things but with ideas about things. Conflicts between people are really conflicts between belief systems. Change *nothing* but the belief and the conflict disappears. Erase the imaginary lines in the earth that separate one nation from another and you have erased nationalistic hostilities. Once we realize that we live in an idea of existence based on no intrinsic realness, we can erase the imaginary line in our minds that separates health and sickness.

We are a species of creature that transforms thought into object. Everything created by humans—from a garden to a cellular phone and the Olympic games—first was a thought. Timothy Ferris, author of *The Mind's Sky*, puts it this way: "We are confronted then, not with the real universe, which remains an eternal riddle, but with whatever model of the universe we can build within the mind."[68] Sandra Ray, author of *Loving Relationships*, says, "If you believe that thought is creative, then you can save yourself." Ralph Waldo Emerson says, "Live with the privilege of Immeasurable Mind." And he also says, "A man is just about as happy as he makes up his mind to be." The same is true of health.

The placebo effect is the effect upon the body of a mind that has been tricked into believing that something outside itself is beneficial or detrimental. The external agent—the crystal or the scalpel—is the rabbit in the hat; the mind is the magician that "doeth the work." If a doctor in whom you had confidence told you he found an infallible soporific that enables chronic insomniacs to sleep all night and you believed him, a water capsule would put you to sleep.

If a placebo can cure you, what has made you sick?

10

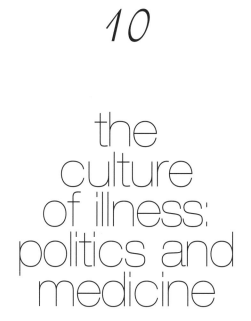

the
culture
of illness:
politics and
medicine

A society constructs the reality it lives in.
—Robert A. Hahn

The total cost of my alternative cancer treatment—
consisting of one intake and one exit interview, a variety
of lab tests, and less than $100 worth of vitamin and
mineral supplements—came to about $500. My insurer,
Community Mutual Blue Cross and Blue Shield of Ohio,
refused to pay for the doctor visits, the supplements, and

some of the laboratory work. In vain I wrote, pointing out the financial disadvantage to their own company of their inflexible coverage policy. They would have had to pay many thousands for the surgery, hospital stay, chemotherapy, and radiation if I had gone that route, yet they denied reimbursement for alternative medicine, which was a fraction of the cost. Medicaid and Medicare take the same illogical position.

Many patients of the MD I went to reported similar experiences with Blue Cross and other health care insurers. One patient was a man whom a conventional doctor had recommended for bypass surgery of four blocked arteries, but instead he elected chelation therapy—the infusion of an amino acid into the bloodstream—which unblocks arteries and clears the blood of heavy metals. His choice, like mine, saved the insurance company many thousands of dollars, yet they rejected his claim for the few hundred spent on chelation.

Similar cases abound. Of the $14 billion spent on alternative medicine in 1990, $10 billion was not covered by insurance companies and had to be paid directly by the patients. Insurance companies typically cover only chiropractic, and even that is a relatively new concession to the burgeoning field of sports medicine. The corporate medical director at Blue Cross, Dr. David Chellappa, offers a strange bit of reasoning to justify his company's refusals: "Things that don't cost a lot aren't worth insuring. A walk every day is good for you, but the employer doesn't pay for it."[69] It's probably futile to point out to Dr. Chellappa that (1) foresighted employers do indeed pay for what's good for their employees by installing running tracks, swimming pools, and nautilus equipment, and (2) employers pay premiums to the insurance company no matter what form of treatment their employees use. It is the insurance company that, having received the premiums, refuses to pay for alternative medicine.

A more sensible argument than Chellappa's might be that unconventional therapies and practitioners are not regulated by the state; therefore, presumably, they are unsafe and ineffective. It would be difficult to measure the relative safety and effectiveness of many alternative medicines, but we do know this: Conventional, regulated medicine is rife with unscrupulous practices, unsafe and unneeded procedures, and—judging by the plethora of victorious malpractice suits—treatments that maim or kill.

I certainly don't recommend banishing government regulation of conventional medicine. We need more rather than less stringent overseeing of the medical and drug industries. But the regulations that now exist do little more than protect the incomes and prestige of MDs. The American Medical Association is as powerful a lobby as the National Rifle Association, and as vigilant in protecting the industry it represents.

We need a watchdog less friendly to these industries. When we learn that in 1994, out of a budget of $11 billion, the National Institutes of Health allocated a paltry $1 million for research into alternative modes—for the entire country, thirty grants of $30,000 each—we have to suspect witting or unwitting government complicity with the medical establishment.

On the surface, it would appear that the situation is

improving: The NIH established an Office of Alternative Medicine (OAM) "to evaluate and determine the efficacy of various unconventional, alternative, and complementary medical practices." The OAM admitted, "There are few research databases which allow for systematic review or meta-analysis of treatment efficacy." Therefore it "feels it is important to better understand if any of these therapies benefit the patients that use them." Notice that the OAM does not see its mission as an investigation into how these therapies benefit patients, but rather if they do. To accomplish this stupendous goal, they offer post-doctoral researchers grants that range from $16,800 to $32,300. Since NIH grants to individuals in conventional fields can run to hundreds of thousands of dollars, one can surmise that applicants will not stampede to research alternative medicine.

If those figures cause skepticism about the sincerity and depth of government interest in alternative medicine, the skepticism may continue despite the formation in 1999 of yet another agency to deal with nonconventional medicine, the National Center for Complementary and Alternative Medicine (NCCA). The NCCA budget for 2001 is $72 million. The NIH budget for the same year is close to $19 billion! Furthermore, the negligible 2.5 percent allowed for research into alternative medicine includes "complementary medicine," which, after all, is nothing more than the introduction of some alternative techniques into a completely orthodox medical model.

When the government encourages people to seek medical attention for present or predicted diseases, its intentions may be laudable. Nevertheless, government programs often result in windfall profits for doctors. For example, in 1976 the Centers for Disease Control issued frightening warnings of a swine flu epidemic of holocaust proportions. As a result, 46 million people were vaccinated—and at $20 a shot—almost $1 billion was transferred from the pockets of the people to the pockets of the vaccine manufacturers and the doctors. No swine flu appeared, but some people died from the vaccination itself.

The intentions of those who propose a national health care plan may also be laudable, but lacking such a program, an estimated 40 million people who are presently uninsured think twice about visiting a doctor and tend to their minor problems themselves. If health care were free, hangnails would be an illness. A national health care plan would generate huge new profits for the medical industry at the same time as it would intensify the "sickness consciousness" of the nation.[70]

A "sickness-conscious society" is, in Ivan Illich's words, "a glaring example of political misuse of scientific achievement to strengthen industrial rather than personal growth. Such medicine is but a device to convince those who are sick and tired of society that it is they who are ill, impotent, and in need of technical repair." The "device" is innocently perpetuated by people who have themselves been snared by the pervasive influence of the medical industry. For example, take my three-year-old granddaughter's book, *Baby Bop Pretends*. The book continues the corruption of my granddaughter's mind that began at her birth. The picture book introduces tots to a variety of people's occupations—teachers, dancers, firefighters, and others—by describing what they do. What it says about doctors is not that they examine you, not that they give you medicine: It says, "Doctors *make* you healthy." They don't "see" if you are healthy. They don't even "keep" you healthy—which might imply that you are already healthy. They *make* you healthy—which of course implies that you are or certainly will be sick, and that a doctor may save you.

⁂

The government's attitude toward faith healing is more overtly antagonistic than its attitude toward alternative medicine. The literature of religious groups, the Christian Science *Chronicle* or *Sentinel*, for example, contains testimonies of hundreds of people who have been healed without medical intervention. Yet neither the medical establishment nor the government has attempted a systematic "scientific" investigation of the validity of these claims. Quite the opposite. Christian Scientists and other faith healers are often prosecuted. When faith healing practiced on a child doesn't work, the entire society feels outrage and the government brings criminal charges against the parents or the faith healer.[71] Headlines scream, "In Treating Sick Children, Prayer Is Not Enough!" "Child Dies Without Medical Treatment!" No headline ever proclaims, "Conventional Medical Treatment Administered: Child Dies!"

If criminal charges are laid upon people whose children die after using faith healing, why aren't criminal charges laid upon doctors whose child patients die in the course of conventional treatment? The answer of course is that the state, with its vast armamentarium of money, law, and the media, fully supports conventional medicine and holds it to be right and good, whereas heterodox healing methods are held to be wrong and bad, deserving of only token funding from government agencies.

Together, government, doctors, pharmaceutical companies, and insurance companies create a cultural mindset that is almost impossible to break out of. The state does not give economic preference to one religion over another, but it does supply huge funds for a certain type of medical treatment. Our democracy has separation of church and state; but, there is no separation of medicine and state.

At the same time, there has never been a more thorough separation of church and health. Healing is completely secularized, and doctors are invested with the power once bestowed upon priests, prophets, and shamans. Patients are expected to comply with the physician's pronouncements; those who do not comply are "wrong" or "bad"[72] and, I might add, exceedingly rare. When Dr. Herbert Benson encouraged one of his patients to pray, the man answered that he had often wanted to pray but felt silly. "Now that you as a doctor say its okay, I'll do it," he said.

Medical practice in every society is "ethnomedicine"—which means that medical practice differs from culture to culture. Yet each culture believes its way is universally right and true. In America, the AMA identifies who is a doctor, designates in what settings medicine is practiced, and even defines what constitutes an illness.

We consider the medicine of primitive cultures to be steeped in magic and superstition; we can't see, because we are immersed in it, the magic and superstition in our own culture. For example, we can't see that our faith in a doctor is responsible for his or her effectiveness. But what, other than the doctor's ability to instill faith, can account for one doctor's great success and another doctor's many failures when both doctors use identical procedures and identical medications in identical offices?

Ideas about health are as sociocentric as ideas about beauty. Particular illnesses are unknown in particular societies, not because the people eat blubber or rice or drink red wine, but because the disease is not important in the cultural consciousness. A disease proliferates when fear of it spreads. In our society, a small segment of the medical profession recognizes, though seldom admits, this biopsychosocial model of illness. But although this segment sees that the culture can exacerbate an illness, or color the patient's view of it, it does not see the culture as the very source of the illness.[73] Nor does it see how government colludes with industry to maintain this cultural mirage.

What you deem to be a disease, the healing method you adopt, and your belief in or despair of recovery are linked to the beliefs of your society. Like all beliefs, they tend to fulfill themselves. In eighteenth- and nineteenth- century England, for example, people were terrified of the weather. "Catching a chill" brought dire consequences. Being caught in the rain was as frightening as if daggers were dropping from the sky. Victorians might have kept "frail" children indoors for an entire winter. Written into the culture was a belief that cold air and rain caused illness, and if accounts in novels and biographies are to be believed, they did. In another culture at another time—in today's America, for example—children play in the snow in tennis shoes and sweaters and splash gaily in downpours without getting sick.

Subconsciously we know that health lies in our own hands. We say things like, "I'd better buy health insurance or I'll certainly get sick," as though the mere possession of health insurance operates like a magic wand to ward off illness. Lacking health insurance, we often do get sick: We worry ourselves into illness.

Governments and social institutions are both the perpetrators and the victims of ideas entrenched in the culture, just as a family may be both perpetrator and victim of ideas handed down through generations of that family. More than we realize, our society promotes "sickness consciousness." The dogmas of the medical industry saturate our thinking. It insists: (1) At one time or another, we are bound to be sick; illness is an *inevitable* component of being alive. (2) Certain ages *inevitably* correlate with certain malfunctions and disease.

That we are a society permeated by health concerns is evident even in our architecture. Our grandest new architecture is not cathedrals or state houses, but medical complexes—the Cleveland Clinic, the Blue Cross building, the sprawling Johns Hopkins compound. The church on every corner has been replaced by medical specialty shops: foot clinics, sleep clinics, diabetes clinics, kidney stone clinics, and instant-care clinics.

Anyone who has somehow broken out of the cultural mindset and believes in psychic healing of any variety faces ridicule. Such a person who happens to be a doctor keeps his or her belief secret and advises patients on the sly that they might try meditation or prayer. The doctor who admits these beliefs openly risks public censure, being shunned by other doctors, and an end to referrals.

The placebo effect must prove to even the most resistant antagonist that, in some cases at least, the mind alone is responsible for producing a physiological effect. But the whole aim in the advertising of drugs, hospitals, doctors, and procedures is to convince the public that everything but the mind is the source of healing. This pernicious advertising is a major player in the culture of illness. It gives the consumer an illusion of choice, but all the competitors play in the establishment arena: Conventional medicine competes with conventional medicine, not with faith or self-healing—just as Coke doesn't compete with water, but with Pepsi. The circle is vicious. We are bombarded on every side with statements that inculcate faith in conventional medicine. Then we are told that we have faith because it works. The fact is, it works because we have faith.

No economic system is more perfect than that of the health industry. The product it sells appears to be doctors, procedures, and various technologies. But those are the *tools* that make the product, not the product itself. The real product the medical industry sells is your well self. The consumer of this product is your sick self or your afraid-you-will-be-a-sick self. You hold the very curious position of being both product and consumer. Health advertising always exploits this double function of yours: It scares you to death and promises salvation at the same time. As long as the industry can generate fear, it creates consumers. Simultaneously, it creates the product. As long as the industry can inspire faith in its tools, the market for product is endless. Both sides precisely match—there is never a surplus of consumers or a shortage of product, because they are one and the same.

Let me end this chapter with a statistic that again illustrates the power that medicine exerts on our thoughts. Women are encouraged to have a mammogram every year after their 50th birthday, and most women obediently trot to the X-ray lab, even though radiation from the X ray itself has been suspected of triggering aberrant cell growth, and even though only 2 or 3 cases are found out of every 1,000 routine mammograms. Presently a strong effort is being made to convince women to have an annual mammogram 10 years earlier—at age 40. The question left unanswered is, what is the sense of a yearly screening when a cancer can take only days or weeks to become detectable? To detect incipient cancers, a woman would need to have a mammogram, not every year, but every month! Other diagnostic cancer tests are equally useless. The positive predictive value of pap smears or of examining the feces

for invisible traces of blood is between 1 and 10 percent
—that is, of every 100 "positive" results, 90 to 99 are
false positives.[74] Yet the very insistence that these tests are
essential, the dire warnings that without them we might
die, keeps us in a subliminal state of fear and tension
that does much to bring on the disease itself.

What is the correlation between the treatment and
the cure of any malady? We are taught to believe that
when we are cured, the drug or the doctor is the direct
cause. But that is only one possible explanation. Two
others are equally logical: nature and the placebo effect.
It is *natural* for the body to heal itself, to avail itself of
"the spontaneous improvement . . . that would have
taken place in the absence of any intervention, the *vis
medicatrix naturae*" —which has been "a most faithful ally
of the medical profession throughout the ages."[75] And
then, there is the placebo effect, the effect that has no
external cause, the effect that is *belief manifested in the
body*. The culture of illness suppresses these truths about
health.

11

propaganda for illness

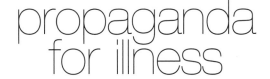

*Most people would prefer risking nuclear annihilation
than risking a fundamental change of mind.*
— *Willis Harman*

If the term "miracle" can apply to anything in my
case, it would not be to my physical healing but to the
opening of my mind. From the time I was a baby, I, like
most of the rest of us in this society, was taught that my
body possessed a threatening life of its own: It became
sick when germs invaded or when ancestors passed on
recalcitrant genes or when, unaccountably, it began
treacherously to malfunction on its own. Except for vac-
cinations, flu shots, and a few drugs that might amelio-
rate the villainy of my forebears, I learned that I would
be powerless against these onslaughts. My blood, liver,

spleen, and heart were fearsome objects that might turn on me at any moment. When they did, doctors and their medicines would be my only hope of salvation.

I was raised in an irreligious home, and nothing in my world—not my friends or my school, not the nature museum, art museum, science museum, movies, newspapers, or magazines—suggested to me a different way of thinking about the health of my body, let alone the possibility that my mind might be involved. A bit of advice about good nutrition was mixed into the medical model, but the advice was mostly wrong. The picture that hung in my second grade classroom, etched even now in my brain, showed the "ideal" meal of meat, milk, butter and white bread, a piece of fruit, and a small portion of vegetable.

Children raised in homes where religion acknowledged such a thing as miraculous healing were certainly not taught that such miracles could happen to them. God perhaps aided, but did not replace, the doctor, who was dependable and could be propitiated with $25. Except for Christian Science and a few minor "cults," religions grant the medical establishment far more power than they grant God. The Catholic Church, for example, recognizes only 64 bona fide miracles to have occurred among the millions of people who have visited Lourdes and among the many hundreds who have testified to their own miraculous healing.

When I became older, I heard of psychosomatic illness, but it was characterized as non-illness invented by mentally ill people. I also heard of spontaneous remissions, but everyone seemed to be dubious of their authenticity, or else dismissed them as inconsequential exceptions. And I heard of placebo effects, but these, too, were shrugged off with phrases like, "It's *only* a placebo effect." People who experienced placebo effects must be a little soft in the head, for how else could they allow a sugar pill to cure their bursitis?

There are disturbed people who cannot stop themselves from running up and down the stairs until they drop from exhaustion, or who check endlessly to see if the oven is off, or who wash their hands to rawness. We recognize obsessive behavior as mental illness. What we don't recognize is that every society produces in its members an obsessive condition of mind that locks them into the ambient ethos. In our society, our minds are saturated with concern for our bodies. We think obsessively about our health. Only when the obsession becomes institutionable—clinical hypochondria or anorexia, for example—do we become aware of it, and then it is an affliction of "those" people, not us.

At a semiconscious level, we live in a constant state of tension with our bodies: "I want to eat but I shouldn't eat" (or shouldn't eat this); "I am too fat" (or too flabby); "I have a headache" (or a knee ache or a neck ache); "I should exercise" (or work out or walk or run); "My hands are chapped" (or I have pimples or freckles); "I am constipated" (or have diarrhea or gas or heartburn); "I have an itchy scalp" (or groin or anus); "I must have an ulcer" (or high blood pressure, or hypoglycemia); and on and on.

Schools, family, friends, the government, and the

media bombard us with reasons to worry: Examine your breasts. Observe your stools. Don't disregard the sneeze or the sniffle—they might harbinger tuberculosis or a fatal pneumonia. Don't ignore the stitch in your side or the pain in your stomach—they might be evidence of . . . ! But thank God, your doctor said to try Mylanta.

As much TV time is devoted to our physical condition as to sex, crime, or sports. Illness is presented regularly as a subtheme in sitcoms and crime shows, and as a major theme in prime-time dramas such as "911" or "ER." People who have courageously endured or bravely died from a whole spectrum of diseases become the heroes of docudramas and documentaries. Endless reels of commercials for pain pills, itch creams, so-called healthful foods, hospitals and clinics, and medical insurance don't let us forget that suffering can begin at any moment.

On one day alone, I saw a program on women's health in general, another specifically on breast cancer, another sponsored by JAMA,[76] 15 advertisements for drugs, 10 advertisements for hospitals, and 7 advertisements for workout machines. And I was watching sporadically, randomly selecting channels, so you can multiply my tally by about 12 hours and 30 or more channels. No commercial told me I could be healthy without hospitals and drugs. Indeed, who would pay for a commercial that had nothing to sell?

In short, during my entire life until January 26, 1982, I had been trained—as all of us are—to think that my body had a kind of independent existence that would be my nemesis. The writing on every wall said, "Expect to be sick."

The mass hypnosis induced by continuous repetition of illness propaganda would be less dangerous if fear and anxiety were all it promoted: More invidious is its message that sickness is somehow desirable. Programs such as ER, the latest and goriest of a long trend from "Marcus Welby, MD" to "Medicine Woman"—convince Americans that illness is inevitable and deliver the appalling idea that sickness makes life interesting.

In these stories, sickness removes patients and their families from the humdrum of everyday life and transforms them into nearly mythical figures engaged in a struggle between the forces of good and the forces of evil. The boredom of routine is replaced by the excitement of crisis. Ordinary, anonymous people become the center of ardent concern. Doctors, nurses, lovers, family, and bystanders all unite in a drama starring the patient. The sick person may have been poor, but now multi-million-dollar equipment serves him; the person may have been unknown, but now the most famous of physicians stands in attendance; the person may have been abused or unloved or ignored, but now the unloving parent or the abusive spouse cries and prays and brings flowers.

How can health and well-being compete theatrically with this melodrama? Health and well-being are happily dull—no plot, no tension, no conflict, and no conquest.

Mary Baker Eddy claimed that the negative thoughts of one person could invade the mind of another and foster "suspicious distrust where honor is due, fear where courage should be strongest, reliance where there should be avoidance, a belief in safety where there is most danger; and these miserable lies, poured constantly into his mind fret, and confuse it."[77] From Franz Mesmer, Eddy adopted the appellation animal magnetism for this invasion. Modern psychiatrists, for example R.D. Laing, or psychologist John Bradshaw, recognize a similar influence and name it "mystification." Children, especially, are spellbound by their family's peculiar ways of looking at things, and get hemmed about with family secrets and deceptions. We, as members of a "culture family," are constantly being mystified in the same way. We think the thoughts of the society—"Eat hamburgers," "Drink Coke," "See a doctor"—and we think they are our own thoughts.

Fortunately, propaganda is never total, even in a totalitarian society—and we live in a relatively free one: There is always some voice in the wilderness that speaks a different truth. Actually, many such voices, if we would only listen for them, throw suspicion on the purported accomplishments of orthodox medicine.

Here are a few examples of deviant messages that might give the thoughtful person pause: Claims have been made that the survival rate (note, not "recovery" rate) for Hodgkin's disease is usually good for patients whose disease is caught early. In the 1940s, the five-year survival rate was 25 percent. By the 1970s, the five-year survival rate rose to 54 percent. Doctors asserted that the increase was due to early detection and chemotherapy.[78] But how can such an assertion be made? The 1940s estimate presumes that every person with Hodgkin's disease sooner or later visited a doctor and that only 25 percent of these patients survived. But what if in the 1940s only half the people with Hodgkin's ever saw a doctor, while the other half were cured either by some other means or, not being "early detected," never knew they had the disease. Let's do the arithmetic: In 1940, 200 people have Hodgkin's. Of these, 100 people do not know they have it, do not feel very ill, and do not go to doctors. They continue with their normal lives, and no medical record includes them. Another 100 become quite ill and do visit doctors. This hundred is treated for the disease, and 25 of those treated live for five years. In this scenario, out of the original 200, 125 live for five years. Now, let's say that in 1970 there are again 200 people with Hodgkin's. By this time, widespread propaganda has convinced people that early detection will save their lives, so 150 of the 200 (plus another 500 who do not have Hodgkin's but fear they do) consult with doctors at the smallest symptom. There are 50 of these 150 who, after chemotherapy, survive for five years. That is a total of only 100 survivors out of 200. Yet, because the statistics include only doctors' patients, the claim can be made that the survival rate has increased by 25 percent.

This kind of distortion of reality is unavoidable given our present assumptions that anyone who is sick sees a doctor. Medical statistics should come with a caveat like cigarette packages: "Warning. These statistics apply only to those people who have visited doctors." The "victory over disease" afforded by early detection may be a complete illusion.

Another reason to suspect the claims of conventional medicine is its inability to discover the causes of most diseases. What passes for a cause is often only the naming of a symptom. "What are these rings around my eyes, doctor?" "They are a collection of dark pigmentation." "Why does my heart race and skip a beat, doc?" "Because you have cardiac arrhythmia."

And what passes for an answer often only begs the question, "What made it go away?" "You've had a spontaneous remission," the doctor solemnly intones.

Isn't there boundless reason to be suspicious of medicine's current truths when medical books become obsolete every few years? Not long ago, six weeks of absolute bed rest was prescribed for myocardial infarction. Now they get "infarcts" up the next day. Not long ago, low roughage diet was prescribed for diverticulitis. Now, high roughage is the standard treatment. Most treatments of cancer include the removal of the tumor at the primary site, and as you know, I myself had a lumpectomy. Now, medical studies say that the cancer at the primary site emits an enzyme that combats the proliferation of cancer cells at further sites—that is, the enzyme inhibits metastasis. But other studies still indicate just the opposite: "We have learned over the years that the remote foci of cancers sometimes regress spontaneously if we surgically remove the primary cancer."[79]

Shouldn't we be suspicious of conventional medicine when an article in the British medical journal *Lancet* presents the following incredible finding: In the 18 developed countries studied, "There is a strong positive association between mortality in children and the *prevalence* of doctors."[80] (Italics mine.) In other words, the more doctors, the higher the death rate. In the face of data like this, who would be so ready to believe the claims of the medical industry were it not for its gigantic public relations effort?

In many respects we Americans are all "from Missouri," but it seems that medicine tends to escape our natural skepticism. Doctors benefit from their patients' illness, not from their wellness. Our national budget and our natural health both would be enormously improved if we could find a way to pay doctors for the absence of sickness.

A person who suffers from rapid heartbeat can take a pill that slows the beat; a yogi can achieve the same result by mental power. Until quite recently, this ability of yogis was denounced as fraudulent. The medical establishment insisted it is impossible to consciously alter the unconscious processes of the body's autonomic system— our blood flows, our heart beats, our temperature rises and falls independently of our mind. Convinced by the doctors, the general public met contrary claims with contempt. Later, when a multitude of studies proved that yogis can at will raise or lower their body temperature, or speed up or slow down their heart rate, doctors were forced to accede to the facts—but they weren't forced to see the importance of the facts.

We, as a society, don't know what to do with the yogis' skill because it runs contrary to our dominant ethos, that is, our belief that mind and body are distinctly separate components of the human being. The mind deals with things invisible—with morals, with realms of the imagination. The body deals with things material and is a material thing—a kind of machine or clock composed of separate parts that have specialized functions.

The God of the mind is somewhere unearthly; the god of the machine is a doctor. He is the mechanic or the clock fixer who adjusts the gears and wheels, and he is as separate from the machine as the machine is from the intangible other part of the human duality, called mind.

The machine metaphor I am using is hackneyed, yet undeniably we do give our body over to others to fix as though it were a machine. We pay to get our bodies off our own hands, even when the hands we deliver ourselves into are also broken. We give our emotions to psychologists who are suicidal, our hearts to obese surgeons, our skin to dermatologists with rashes. One of the many lectures on health I attended was given by a doctor who spoke about the amazing benefits of vegetarianism and acupuncture. She spoke from a wheelchair and suffered from arthritis so severe that an attendant had to hold the microphone, yet many in the audience found in her illness no contradiction and were ready to trust her recommendations.

Our society pays dearly for our preoccupation with our bodies. It pays in the form of ill health, and it pays in the form of dollars—more than a trillion of them. In 1998, health care cost us $1.15 billion! The debate about whether we should institute a national health care program is largely a debate about money. No side in the debate takes the position that perhaps illness needn't be ubiquitous and inevitable, or that a medical elite needn't be called upon to cure a population of helpless consumers. This controversy leaves out a crucial fact: In 80 percent of illnesses, the doctor is nature. As one doctor points out, "The patient is rarely introduced to this bene-factor—an *éminence grise* who is consulted in secret."

We pay stupendous amounts to cure illnesses which if left alone would cure themselves. Medicine is literally the only profession that we monetarily compensate for a result that would take place anyway in the course of a few days. Wouldn't gardeners love to be paid for lawns that mowed themselves, or beauticians for hair that styled itself? When insurance, either private or govern-mental, pays the bill and when people are fixated on the state of their bodies, they will run to doctors with sniffles and paper cuts or, routinely, with nothing.

Health is available to everyone and costs little. It doesn't depend upon new therapeutic techniques or new technologies, but upon a change of mind about *who is in control*. It depends upon the willingness of people to engage in self-care. If ever you have had an illness that automatically improved, you have demonstrated your power to heal yourself. If ever you have had a placebo heal you, you have demonstrated that the power resides in your mind.

A linguistic theory called the Sapir-Wharf Hypoth-esis says that perception is structured by language: We do not become aware of something until we have a name for it. A corollary to this theory says that we are deceived into seeing something that is not there when we do have a name for it. The vocabulary of faith and self-healing is pitifully meager; it comes from the scanty lexicon of mysticism and metaphysics. The vocabulary of medicine is enormous; volumes of terms name procedures, conditions, and cures. And as I have shown, the rhetoric that persuades us to trust doctors and hospitals and to fear illness and disease is endless. This language is a cultural sleight-of-hand, an abracadabra that tricks us into believing that sickness is within our bodies and sooner or later must show up.

In a story by Nancy Willard, "Things Invisible to See," the heroine, a lame girl named Clair, has a medical epiphany—one that our whole society would be blessed to experience. She sees that the doctors and nurses "were not healing her. They were teaching her to take her place among the handicapped."

12

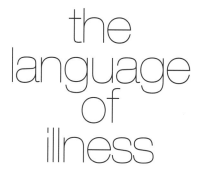

the language of illness

*Mankind in all ages has had a strong propensity
to conclude that wherever there is a name, there
must be a distinguishable separate entity
corresponding to the name.*

—*John Stuart Mill*

Is it possible that people who are diagnosed with
cancer die of a sophisticated form of voodoo? Does the
victim's *belief* in the power of vicious cells, like *belief* in
the power of a hex, lead to his death? "Cancer" is a
demon word—the destructiveness of cancer begins as
soon as the diagnosis is uttered. The dread label starts a

Rube Goldberg reaction: The word strikes terror to the heart; terror releases gushes of adrenaline; the outpouring of adrenaline upsets normal biological functions and weakens the immune system; and the weakened immune system permits cancer cells to proliferate. The word, we are incessantly warned, demands immediate action, and so terrified patients place themselves in the hands of physicians who insult their already fear-damaged bodies by attacking them with chemotherapy and radiation.

The urgent extremes of cancer treatment are based on a commonly held and, some doctors believe, false understanding of its nature. These doctors maintain that cancer cells are systemic, that all of us are developing and ridding ourselves of cancer cells all the time, and that "our body defenses recognize them, attack them and take care of the matter."[81] But most doctors disregard this evidence that cancer cells come and go; rather they view cancer as a localized cluster of cells gone crazy.

The role of the individual is very different in these two formulations. If we are developing cancer cells all the time, then we can control them in the same way we do cuts and bruises—by the body's natural healing processes. But if cancer is a berserk bunch of wildly proliferating cells that seem to have a mind of their own, we need to hire mercenaries to help fight the battle. The language associated with cancer, the metaphors used to describe the disease, engrave it in our minds as a spreading spider's web or an omnivorous octopus that invades and engulfs.

Words act as powerful placebos in all diseases, not just cancer. They also act as powerful nocebos—that is, they can produce deleterious rather than salutary effects. ("Nocebo" is a word coined to contrast with placebo. It means "to harm" rather than "to please.") A good example of the way words alone can affect the course of a disease and its treatment is found in the case of hyperparathyroidism, a disorder in the regulation of blood calcium. The disorder is seldom life-threatening and—while most doctors would recommend removal of the thyroid if the malfunction is severe—its mild form is hardly worth troubling with. Until multiple-component blood testing became part of routine examinations, the disease was rarely detected. Since testing became routine, however, surgical removal of the thyroid is almost standard treatment. The large number of patients who had a mild, previously undetected condition and were undergoing surgery prompted an investigation by the Mayo Clinic.

The investigation revealed that the mere naming of a disease is a more powerful indicator of treatment than the disease itself: One group, randomly selected, was assigned for immediate surgery. The other group was told they had mild hyperparathyroidism and that surgery was available if they desired, but was not essential and was not assigned. Yet each and every person in the second group elected to have surgery! Telling them they had the condition actually made the condition worse or made the person perceive it as worse. As one of the investigators pointed out, "The anxiety of having a disorder that could be surgically treated was simply too discomforting"[82]—never mind that the risks attending anesthesia and surgery were greater than the risks of mild hyperparathyroidism.

Linguists have identified phenomena that they refer to as "verbal realism" and "symbol realism." These terms mean that the mind responds to words or iconic objects as strongly as it would to the things they represent. In symbol realism, the sight of a symbolic object, for example the flag of the United States, can evoke patriotic feelings so intense that people are willing to die to protect it—a piece of red, white, and blue cloth, in effect, has become the virtual country. In verbal realism, a word carries the emotional power of the real thing. A person uttering an ethnic slur, like "nigger," for example, can arouse as much anger as if the speaker had actually assaulted an African American. "Nigger" or "kike" or "wop" takes on a life of its own and causes a bio/emotional reaction: "Them's fight'n words," as our Western heroes say. Apply this language phenomenon to the area of health, and you can see that a word or symbol can make you ill.

Language used as an instrument of power is probably coeval with language itself. The magician, standing within the magic circle, can summon by incantation the powers that will cure or kill. In some cultures, one's true name must not be spoken, as one's soul would escape on the breath that carries the word. In many religions, speaking the name of a god captures the essence of that god and brings him forth. Among Jews, on the other hand, God's name must not be pronounced, for saying the name would defile him.

In Judaism, the most potent words are found in the Torah where God himself connects his words with healing: "If thou wilt diligently hearken to the voice of the Lord thy god, and wilt do that which is right in His eyes, and wilt give ear to His commandments and keep His statutes, I will put none of the diseases upon thee which I have put upon the Egyptians: for I am the Lord that healeth thee."[83]

When Jesus cured the blind man at Bethsaida, he knew that it was imperative to keep him away from the society of those who believed in and spoke of disease. After the man's blindness was healed, Jesus instructed him not to return to the village, but to go directly to his own home.

Origen, a church father of the second century, asserted that a successful exorcism did not depend on the Lord Himself. Origen taught that the magical potency resided in the letters of the name—J-E-S-U-S.

The language of medicine has a profound effect upon the practice of medicine. As far back as can be traced, physicians have recognized that merely to name a disease, merely to prescribe a remedy, merely to don medical vestments, causes something to happen in the body of the patient.

In our society, scientific terms are magical. Call an over-the-counter allergy pill "anistophymilycin" and you give it the enhanced healing power of a prescription drug. Doctors have empowered placebos by calling them by names that sound scientific, such as "tincture of Condurango" or "fluid-extract of Cimicifuga nigra."

If language, by its effect upon mind, causes prejudice against a race or a gender; if the words used to describe people, such as "cripple," "snot-nosed kid," and "bimbo," influence our behavior toward them; if spreading the word that a company's stock is valuable can raise the price of that stock regardless of the peform- ance of the company; if the scent of a woman's perfume in a room after the woman has exited can produce not only amorous feelings but even an erection—how can we refuse to see that words and symbols create our concepts about health and illness, and that these concepts affect our health? If we do refuse to see this fact, it proves that our mindset is influenced by the spell of language more in the domain of medicine than elsewhere.

Scientists focus on the physical world largely because only physical phenomena can be measured, regulated, and duplicated. The effects of symbols cannot be controlled. The effects of symbols are attached to the unique situation and the unique individual: Emotions a person may feel when he sees the American flag will be different today than tomorrow, and different at a US post office than in a foreign country. Symbols are the prover- bial river that cannot be stepped into twice. Yet the effect of any given symbol on the biology of any given human is as real as anything science can reproduce in a con- trolled study.

If a woman doesn't eat because the word "fat" and the symbolism of fatness terrify her, she is as skinny as if she had cancer of the stomach. Because control and replication are requisites of the scientific method, science dismisses as unreal or untrue empirical evidence that can be *verified* but not precisely *duplicated*—that is, science dismisses the empirical evidence of practically everything in life. To paraphrase Lao-Tzu, "If you can name it, it isn't that." I might add, "If you can prove it in the laboratory, it isn't so."

Someone said, "Diseases that do not have names do not exist." The fearsome corollary to that observation is that diseases can be made to exist by naming them. In 1975, Agence France-Presse carried a report on a disease called *Koro,* a Javenese word meaning "the head of the turtle." The disease was attributed to eating "tunny fish" and was supposed to cause the penis to wither. The disease spread to Malaysia and south China where it was known as *Shook Yang,* (shrinking penis).[84] Men afflicted by this malady lived in terror of dying and tried to prevent their penis from disappearing into their abdominal cavity by holding it with clamps, chopsticks, clothes pins, or even safety pins. "In some instances," the French paper reported, "relatives would take turns 'to hold on to the penis,' and sometimes the wife was asked to keep the penis in her mouth to assuage the patient's fear." No one knows the origin of this fictional disease. It was entirely a product of autosuggestion or what Phineas Parkhurst-Quimby and Mary Baker Eddy would have called false belief, yet Koro reached epidemic proportions.

If we are to take our health into our own hands, we need to understand that symbol realism and verbal realism, which have absolutely nothing to do with actuality, permeate medicine. We respect and entrust our healing to the person identified by the rubric "doctor," irrespective of the verifiable and proven healing capabilities of that individual. How many of our "diseases" are "non-diseases," pure figments of the imagination made real by symbols and words? Quimby and Eddy would say all of them.

I don't mean to question the motives of doctors.[85] Certainly many, perhaps most, are devoted to helping others. But we can't disregard the fact that when doctors treat "non-diseases," they reap handsome monetary rewards. There is no profit to be made if there is no treatment. Whether intentionally or not, we are taught that an elite group possesses abilities unavailable to the rest of us, and wampum, greenbacks, cash, or colored beads flow continuously from the helpless to the ones who come to save them.

Our language establishes a materialistic perception of life: "It's all in your mind," we are told, or "It's just your imagination"—meaning of course that whatever it is, it isn't real. How different our lives would be if from earliest childhood we heard that it is all in your mind and that your imagination creates what happens to you. How different our health would be if instead of, "It might be serious, go see a doctor," we were told, "Don't give it a thought, it's only a microbe," or, "Don't waste your time taking medicine, put your mind to it instead, put your imagination to it." If we could think of the words "mind" and "body" as semantic distinctions—not actually two different things—then we would be on the road to life-long health.

Unfortunately, the language available for intelligently describing states of wellness is very spare. We have psychobabble and New Age banalities that really don't help dislodge the semantic system that keeps medicine entrenched in our minds and thereby in our lives. How can we find our way out of the trap of language? This disturbing question may be asked of every culture's values. In America, unlike other far more insular societies, we have access to alternative attitudes and alternative practices that break through the monolith of convention. We can give credence to ideas and testimonies that contradict the rhetoric of organized medicine. "A road is made by people walking on it," says a Zen master.

13

varieties of faith

We have our brush and colors—
paint paradise and in we go.

—*Kazantzakis*

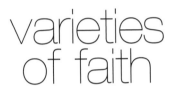

All healing is faith healing. By "faith" I don't mean belief in a set of abstract ideas; I mean belief that motivates action. Faith healing is not necessarily a nonmedical process; it may be a medical process. By my definition, faith is not measured by lip service; *it is demonstrated by how you live.* In regard to health, your true faith is revealed by the type of treatment you choose and the belief that underlies your choice. These are possible varieties:

> 1. Faith in doctors or in alternative medical practitioners and their technologies—as instruments of science

2. Faith in doctors or in alternative medical prac-
   tioners and their technologies—as instruments
   of God

3. Faith in magical objects such as crystals and
   crucifixes—as instruments of God

4. Faith in faith healers, people possessed of
   supernatural powers—as instruments of God

5. Faith in healing that comes without a
   middleman, directly from God

6. Minimal faith in any of these possibilities,
   depending on the mood and the moment

7. Faith in nothing, with the hope, however,
   that although nature is engaged in a constant
   battle with itself, science might tilt the battle
   in the patient's favor

8. Faith in the power of the self to heal the self

Today the largest category seems to be the first:
People have faith in science and technology.

Among people who consider themselves religious or
spiritual, the greatest number would fall into category 2.
They believe that the capabilities of doctors and nature
are endowed by God. An apocryphal book of the Old
Testament says, "Honor a physician with the honor due
unto him for the uses which ye may have of him: for the
Lord hath created him. . . . The Lord hath created medicines out of the earth. . . . Of such doth the apothecary
make a confection." (Wisdom of Jesus, Son of Sirach
38:1.)

Relatively few religious people believe God heals
them directly. Cardiac patient Thomas Canterbury is a
good example of category 5: Three years after his second

heart attack, a heart catheterization indicated his need for bypass surgery, which was duly scheduled. He and his wife prayed, and Thomas says that while they were praying, "a warm feeling . . . flushed throughout my whole body." The following day the coronary specialist told the Canterburys, "Something funny has happened": The coronary arteries on the left side of Thomas's heart remained blocked, but a new vein had grown from the right ventricle to the left side of the heart and was supplying blood.[86]

Yet Canterbury's extraordinary recovery does not stop him from seeking "the best medical attention" when any illness threatens. His irrepressible faith in medicine is a perfect illustration of Philo Judaeus's (30 BCE– 40 CE) comment: "Men do not trust God the Savior completely, but have recourse to the aids which nature offers, doctors, herbs, medicinal compounds and rigid diet."[87]

It seems reasonable to ask why, if a person can grow new veins practically overnight by praying, anyone needs to see a doctor for anything. The same question might be asked of the members of two religious groups that fully accept faith healing—Pentecostals and Catholic Charismatics. Both these religions differ from traditional Christianity in placing paramount importance on direct contact with Jesus. But while Jesus may be utilized to heal, he apparently needs the complement of mainstream medicine. Pentecostals and Charismatics may be "slain in spirit" on Sunday and presumably healed during those moments (sometimes hours) of invasion by the divine, yet on Monday seek medical treatment.

With the exception of Christian Science and, to a lesser extent, some of the other New Age metaphysical religions (e.g., the Unity School of Christianity and the United Church of Religious Science), religious faith does not compete with faith in conventional medicine; it accommodates it. The competition to conventional medicine comes from various alternative medicines, which also compete with each other. Believers in macrobiotic diets challenge believers in raw food diets; believers in TM doubt psychic surgeons, and so on.

Nonmedical healing is seen as miraculous by both mainstream and divergent religions. A miracle is, by definition, divine intervention in human affairs, an effect not expected to happen, a phenomenon not assigned to material cause. A miracle inspires wonder and awe. Healed people feel specially elected to have received such a blessing, and become—both to themselves and others—the stuff that legend and myth are made of.

Self-healing, on the other hand, has none of the grandeur of a miracle. It is a small event that hardly anyone knows about. Faith in self-healing is a lonely faith. There is no glory in self-healing, and no story. The only reward is the cessation of sickness.

Having no church or organization or community of like-minded individuals to support them, the few who believe in the reality of self-healing and try to practice it must summon from somewhere the strength to withstand the beliefs of their society. Support groups, Twelve-Step groups, prayer groups, and healing circles abound for every imaginable physical and emotional problem, as adjuncts to other forms of treatment. To my knowledge, there is no group to support the aim or ease the isolation of self-healers.[88]

Healing a specific ailment depends upon the degree of faith the patient has in the treatment, regardless of what stimulates that faith. *Lasting* health is a different matter, a spiritual matter, and I deal with that in the final chapter of this book.

To me, self-healing is a plain truth. Why is this truth known to so few? The answer is the cultural mystification I spoke of in the preceding chapter. Every culture—secular and religious—singles out only certain things to believe in; and, with few exceptions, the major medical paradigm of every culture places the power of healing in someone or in something outside the self.

But every religion that I know of, from animism to Buddhism, also contains a minor strain of faith in the power of the individual. "Thou art That," says Hinduism. "What I have done, can ye do, and even more than I have done," says Jesus. "The Christ is *in* you," say the New Age religions. "As above, so below," say the occult religions. In Judaism, there is a link between morality and health that suggests that intervention by priest or physician is not only unneeded but may constitute an impiety because health is inherent in virtue, and health is a part of God's design that accompanies righteousness: "My son, in thy sickness be not negligent: but pray unto the Lord and he will make thee whole. Leave off from sin, and order thine hands aright, and cleanse thy heart from all wickedness. . . ."[89]

Theosophy, Christian Science, and Unity—late off-shoots of Christianity blended with other spiritual disciplines—practice what they judge to be the original Christianity of Jesus, and they do emphasize self-healing. In their view, health is built into God's creation, as an integral element. If you are in tune with universal forces, you do not have to work to achieve health any more than you have to work to breathe or to circulate blood; you *will* be healthy if you do not do something to block health. In theory, no object or second person is needed to mediate between the material and the spiritual world: The individual is It. In practice, however, few adherents of these religions replace faith in medicine with faith in their indwelling healer.

Because Christian Science, Theosophy, and Unity—all founded within 50 years of each other—affirm self-healing, it is important to examine their teaching more closely.[90] Unity and Theosophy have antecedents in Rosicrucianism, which grew out of the occult practices of ancient Greece and the Hebrew Kabbala, and also antecedents in Swedenborgianism, which grew out of a revelation of Emanuel Swedenborg in the eighteenth century. All three religions contributed ideas to the spiritual revival of the mid-nineteenth century—The New Thought Movement, or Truth Movement, as it is sometimes called. Figures as different as the poet William

Butler Yeats and the American transcendentalist Ralph Waldo Emerson are associated with New Thought, as are movements as diverse as Vedanta and the Emmanuel movement.

The Church of Christ, Scientist— Christian Science

Christian Science—and, to my knowledge, only Christian Science—teaches self-healing as a definitive dogma. Theosophists as well as members of Unity and the other "science" religions are "allowed" to consult doctors. One congregation may consider this a concession to individuals who have not yet reached a higher state of consciousness, another congregation may hold that God's presence is in everything, including doctors and drugs. Because its fundamental tenet holds that the material world does not exist, Christian Science views medical treatment as an unacceptable compromise. Neither the ailment nor the doctor's treatment is real: There can be no bodily illness because there is no body—both are figments of mind in the same sense that dreams are figments of mind. A dreamed illness is not an illness. (My own belief, which I present in the last chapter of this book, is very similar to Christian Science; yet my belief includes, while Christian Science does not, the ideas of many other teachings—including Unity, Theosophy, Judaism, and Buddhism. More important, I do not deny the existence of the material world, but rather regard spirit and matter as different forms of a single substance.)

Mary Baker Eddy founded Christian Science in Boston in 1867, and for years it was the fastest-growing religion in America. The origin of Christian Science can be traced to Eddy's recovery from a debilitating back problem, under the care of Phineas Parkhurst-Quimby (see chapter 9). Her back problem later returned, and she then cured herself after experiencing a religious epiphany that left no room to doubt the nonphysical origin of physical problems.[91] After the epiphany, she could not believe that such a thing as illness could exist in God's creation: If God is good, she reasoned, then sickness cannot come from God. And because God is the origin of all things, sickness can be nothing more than an illusion: "There is no life, truth, intelligence, nor substance in matter. All is infinite Mind and its infinite manifestation. Spirit is immortal Truth; matter is mortal error. Spirit is the real and eternal; matter is the unreal and temporal."[92]

The metaphysics of Christian Science may be called "objective idealism": "Ideal" because there is "no truth in matter"; "objective" because metaphysical laws are immutable and universal and—like the laws of nature—can be verified objectively.

Christian Science, like Unity and Theosophy, rejects the idea that God favors certain individuals with health and good fortune. Unlike traditional Christianity, no minister or scripture stands between the individual and the divine. The Church of Christ Scientist helps the individual demonstrate his own Christian power, most clearly manifested in self-healing.

Theosophy

Helena Petrovna Blavatsky (1831–1891) founded

the Theosophical Society in 1875. Described by William Butler Yeats as "a sort of old Irish peasant woman with an air of humor and audacious power," she arrived in America in 1873 at age 42, drawn by the enormous popularity of Spiritualism—18 million Americans, almost half the total population, attended séances and read Spiritualist papers.[93]

Blavatsky taught the doctrine of Astral Light—the vital ether that Hindu mystics call by the Sanskrit term *Akasha*. "Theosophy," which means knowledge of God or divine wisdom, teaches that ultimate knowledge is accessible to anyone who has developed a certain quality of consciousness through Akasha. Down through the ages, a secret brotherhood of adepts transmits higher knowledge to those who are ready to receive it.[94]

Theosophy's idea of a sacred brotherhood of unidentified superior beings, the "Masters," is not new or unique. Among other places, it is found in Rosicrucianism, in Swedenborgianism, in Judaism, and in Buddhism. Judaic tradition has it that 36 extraordinary people—pillars of righteousness—(whose identities are hidden) live on Earth at all times; and, through the influence of their spiritual and moral perfection, act as anchors for humanity. Buddhism teaches that enlightened beings, the bodhisattvas, may choose either to enter nirvana or—out of compassion for the unenlightened on Earth—may return to ordinary human existence to help.

Theosophists share with Rosicrucians some of the following beliefs about health: The human body is a force field or energy field. Its limbs and organs connect as if by invisible cables to a vast, intangible world, from which it receives and to which it sends powerful streams of energy. The brain is the efflorescence, the bursting into flower, of the spine. The vertebrae mark the stations of a mystical ladder and form the main channel conducting the downward flow of energy from the mental plexus and the upward flow of energy from the earth.

This interchange between the human body, earth energy, and cosmic energy accounts for self-healing. The feet form the natural point of contact with Mother Earth and conduct earth energy through the body. The hands absorb psychic energy from the space surrounding the body (the "Akashic Envelope"), concentrate it in the palm, and send it by way of the fingers to any place needing to be healed. (Belief in the supernatural power of the hand is actually widespread in both occult and orthodox practices; it is implied in the laying on of hands, in palm reading, and in the gesture of blessing. In ancient Greece, a man with a deformed hand could never hold high office in the priesthood.)

Unity School of Christianity—Unity

Unity is a later development of the American spiritual renaissance of the nineteenth century. Early in the century, American Transcendentalists had introduced Eastern mysticism and caused a great stirring up of America's mostly Protestant, mainly traditional, beliefs. Now hundreds of thousands of people, ranging from the simply curious to serious seekers of a new kind of spirituality, attended lectures on metaphysics and Eastern thought of widely different kinds. Unity was literally born at one of these lectures.

One evening in the spring of 1886, Myrtle Fillmore, an ill woman, attended a lecture given by a Dr. E.B. Weeks, who had been trained by Emma Curtis Hopkins, a former student of Mary Baker Eddy. During the lecture, Myrtle became profoundly convinced that bodily ills generate in the mind. She exited the lecture hall a new woman, repeating to herself, "I am a child of God and therefore I do not inherit sickness." She began to apply metaphysical principles to her illness and to her life in general. And, in two years, she was completely free of the tuberculosis she had suffered since childhood—which, by the night of the lecture, had worsened to a point where doctors predicted imminent death. She wrote: "I want everybody to know about this beautiful, true law, and to use it. It is not a new discovery, but when you use it and get the fruits of health and harmony, it will seem new to you, and you will feel that it is your own discovery."[95]

Unity is extremely eclectic. It propounds no dogma but is held together by two beliefs: that each individual is a Christ and that each individual's life experience is an outpicturing of his or her inner consciousness.[96]

These three religions,[97] while different in many ways, are alike in stressing the nonmaterial dimension of reality, in locating the source of healing in that dimension, and in identifying the mind as the cause of every event. They incorporate teachings from many non–Judeo-Christian religions—Hinduism, Buddhism, Taoism, and Sufism. Theosophy and Unity do this intentionally; and Christian Science does this probably unintentionally.

These religions teach that healing is a practice
of everyday life performed by ordinary people, rather
than associated with special rituals, special training,
or specially gifted persons. They expect faith to prove
itself pragmatically by becoming actual experience.

I don't want to leave this brief overview of the
religions that recognize the power of mind without
mentioning that these ideas show up universally in
literature, too.

The main character in Herman Melville's *The
Confidence Man* is a fraud and an impostor, but he is
able—by mental suggestion—to make others do as he
advises, even when his advice is completely at variance
with their character and usual behavior. Melville
illustrates the latent capacities for good or ill that can
be released when people take an idea to heart.

In one episode, the Confidence Man, disguised as an
herb doctor, offers an herbal remedy ("Omni-Balsamic
Reinvigorator") to an invalid whom science with its
"tinctures and fumes, and braziers" had been unable to
cure. When the sick man inquires about the ingredients
of the Reinvigorator, the Confidence Man admonishes
him for being too analytical, too much a philosopher.
He exhorts the sick man: "Work upon yourself, invoke
confidence, though from ashes; rouse it; for your life,
rouse it, and invoke it, I say." This instruction is
perfectly consistent with the New Thought religions. I am
no materialist, says the Confidence Man, "but the mind
so acts upon the body, that if the one have no
confidence, neither has the other."[98]

The Wizard of Oz is a notable example of the placebo

effect dramatized in literature. Like the Confidence Man, the Wizard is a fraud and a humbug—a bag of wind who, appropriately, once operated a hot-air-balloon concession at a circus. Yet this trickster is able to transform one being with no heart, one with no brain, and one with no courage into the ideal selves each one longs to be. How does he perform these feats? Does he possess supernatural powers, as they believe? Not at all. Their brainless, heartless, spineless behavior had been self-fulfilling prophecies. The great Wizard confesses that he has nothing to give them that they don't already possess, but they disregard his confession. They believe he has the power to transform them, and their belief is the power that works the transformation.[99]

A charlatan and a healer perceive themselves differently: Charlatans know they are deceiving and healers believe they are healing, but to the person who is healed, they are identical.

William Blake is perhaps the premier writer whose work contains the metaphysics of New Thought. His ideas spring from many of the same sources. If Blavatsky, Eddy, and the Fillmores had lived a hundred years earlier, and if they had been incomparable poets, they might have written Blake's prophetic works. He rejected the materialism of Bacon, Newton, and Locke, and countered with the idealism of Plato, Plotinus, and Berkeley, working their metaphysics into an elaborate poetic universe of the mind.

Blake draws a hierarchy of four worlds, which represent states of consciousness: The highest is the world of Imagination. The lowest is the world of discrete material objects. Every person inhabits his own Eden, his "garden on a mount," which is a projection of his own consciousness. In Blake's words: "As a man is, so he Sees. As the Eye is formed, such are its Powers. You certainly mistake, when you say that the Visions of Fancy are not to be found in this World. To Me This World is all One continued Vision of Fancy or Imagination."

Blake speaks of a "new church" that would preach the religion of "God as man" —the "Divine Humanity" present in every individual: in Blake's terms, Jesus the Imagination. This new church sounds much like Unity, and the words Blake uses might well have come out of the mouth of Mary Baker Eddy: "Error is Created. Truth is Eternal. Error, or Creation, will be Burned up, and then, and not till then, Truth of Eternity will appear. It is Burnt up the Moment Men cease to behold it."

The possibility that reality is nothing more than a function of perception is very frightening to most of us. We persist in asking, "But what is *really* real?" How can we conduct our lives if there is no objective reality, no objective truth? Upon what do we build our values, our institutions? Of course the answer is that our values, too, are invented, and our institutions are merely warehouses to contain them. Science, however, steps in to answer the question in its own way, and the idiosyncratic standard of science has become our reality: What is really real, science says, is what we can measure under controlled conditions; the truth is what these measurements disclose.

Many Americans profess to believe in a reality that

transcends the measurable world. In 1992, 50 percent of Americans said they believe in angels, 46 percent in ESP, 37 percent in devils. Among those who hold these beliefs, a disproportionate number are college educated.[100] Today I surmise that these numbers are even higher. Also, college graduates believe in clairvoyance more than those who don't go to college. But how many among these "believers," as well as among Swedenborgians, Theosophists, Anthroposophists, Hindus, Buddhists, Unity, Christian Scientists, Charismatics, and Pentecostals, et cetera, *live* their belief? How many who believe spiritual health exists draw from this spiritual health their physical health?

⌐

I mentioned in chapters 8 and 9 how politically dangerous it has always been to practice religious healing—the practice closest to self-healing—unless it is performed as a supplement to medical healing. Any assertion that contains an error, any failure to perform exactly as promised, is taken as proof of fraud and charlatanism. For example, in 1743, a Freemason, Count Alessandro Cagliostro, was reared a Catholic but was deeply interested in Swedenborg and in magic (for which he found biblical justification in the miraculous powers of Moses, the secrets of King Solomon, prophetic vision, and the witch of Endor). Convinced that, with divine help, heavenly magic could be rediscovered, he established a medical practice in which he accomplished remarkable cures based on this belief. He was attacked by both the medical world, which saw a threat to the profession in the cures he achieved, and the clergy, who saw his "miracles" as a menace to the Church.[101] The same two-flanked attack was waged against Mary Baker Eddy: Establishment medicine vilified her and Protestant ministers condemned Christian Science as a cult.

In our time, establishment medicine has the full force of government and the law to back it up. If you believe in faith healers or believe that healing comes directly from God (categories 4 or 5 as defined above), and if you live by your faith, you could be in serious trouble. In 1984, a Christian Scientist whose four-year-old died of acute bacterial meningitis was blasted by the news media for "murderous neglect," and the court ruled that the mother could be prosecuted for the death of her daughter. In 1986, two-year-old Robin Twitchel died in Boston of a bowel obstruction. The child's Christian Scientist parents and a Christian Scientist practitioner had been praying for her recovery. The parents were convicted of manslaughter for "doing nothing."[102]

But who determines what constitutes "nothing" and what constitutes "something"? If a person has faith in an object or procedure, to that person it is something. To Robin Twitchel's parents, the destructive route would have been medical treatment. It would have been worse than nothing. Unfortunately, Robin Twitchel died; but if death is the measurement of doing nothing, thousands of doctors will be facing prosecution for manslaughter. No wonder doctors conceal their belief in nonmedical approaches. One doctor admits that when he suggests to a hospital patient the possibility of nonphysical sources of healing, he waits until the other doctors have left the room.[103]

Today, those who blaspheme conventional medicine by practicing faith healing aren't burned at the stake, but they are burned in the court of public opinion and are thought to be, at the very least, crazy or idiots.

⌒

The placebo effect is not hypothetical; it has been scientifically demonstrated that healing occurs when one has faith that it will occur. This faith does not have to be linked to any sort of divinity: Faith in the curative power of anything will produce a cure; the more complete the faith, the more complete the cure. Conversely, when faith falters, the curative power of anything declines. When faith healing in the traditional sense is practiced, the power does not reside in the healer but in the subject's faith in the healer. I am not a healer, but if you believe that I can heal you, then I can heal you.

If I *were* to heal you, the healing could not be scientifically proven because it could not be replicated. It could not be replicated because there is not another you, not another identical situation, and not another relationship identical to the one between you and me. But though a particular case cannot not be replicated, the sheer number of particular cases is overwhelming evidence that spontaneous healing does occur. *That* this happens is not in question. The question is what makes it happen. Doctors label the mysterious disappearance of a malady as a "remission" or a placebo effect—which is another way of saying they don't know what made it go away. Traditional religions call such disappearances "miracles."

Each of us lives in a different world, defined by what we have faith in. If you're an atheist, talking to God is a sign either of ignorance or of a mental disorder. If you're religious, God is the best "person" to talk to. Those who believe in scientific medicine, those who believe in religious healing, and the few who believe in self-healing "do not simply see the world differently; they see a different world."[104] The person who sees the cure as existing in penicillin or some other compound simply doesn't comprehend an alternative explanation, even when it would seem glaringly obvious to someone else.

One doctor, for example, demonstrates a great insight when he says, "The pill the patient swallows, no matter what its nature [e.g., sugar water] acquires its potency as a *symbol* of faith, wisdom, and support." Yet this doctor annuls his own insight: "Man in distress wants action—rational action if possible, of course, but irrational action, if necessary, rather than none at all."[105] The irrational action presumably is the sugar pill. But if a doctor has administered a placebo purely to satisfy his patient's desire for action, the patient is not the irrational one, the doctor is. And if the sugar pill acquires potency simply because the patient believes it is a drug, the doctor would be irrational not to administer it.

The factors that inspire faith are different for each person and for the same person at different times, so they cannot be measured in the laboratory. What can be measured in the laboratory is whether a diagnosed disease has disappeared. If we take the whole world as the laboratory and the whole of recorded time as the temporal boundary of the experiment, the placebo effect has been replicated millions of times.

Not so long ago, physicists talked of something called ether; they found it necessary to postulate some kind of material that could conduct visual images and sound waves through space. But there probably is no such thing as ether; physicists invented it. Today, physicists have brought electrons into being: Electrons cannot be apprehended by the senses; they are postulates, created to explain certain physical phenomena. At a Jehovah's Witness service, Jehovah is *no less present* as a real experience to the participants than electrons are to a group of physicists. And a Jehovah's Witness can replicate his experience and prove its effect on his body no less than the physicist can prove the existence of electrons. Which is the fact? The whole history of science is one long correction of "facts."

To hold faith in anything steadily and unwaveringly seems practically impossible. Mystics speak of the dark night of the soul—times when faith slips away. Only the greatest religious figures of human history—Jesus, Buddha, Moses—are unbrokenly faithful. The rest of us slip from even the faith we hold most ardently: An atheist one day prays. A self-healer breaks a leg and visits a doctor. But our doubts and fears do not change the truth: There is only one source of healing, and it is you.

14

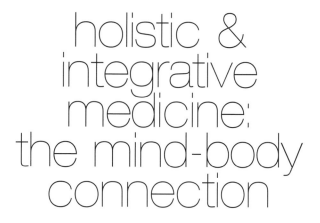

holistic & integrative medicine: the mind-body connection

*We are trained or conditioned to conceive of teachers
as always being outside us.*

— Dr. Brugh Joy

⌒

    All medical schools educate prospective doctors
in the physiology of the brain; few educate them in the
psychology of the mind. However, once out in the real
world of patient care, some doctors learn that the intangible parts of their patients—those parts that cannot be

seen or touched—do bear on the effectiveness of medical treatment. One survey found that once doctors complete their formal training, as they continue to practice, they tend to become more attuned to the importance of what their patients are thinking and feeling: The doctors listen more, they talk more; and they intuit more of what is going on in the patient's unarticulated emotions. In short, what the survey found was a growing awareness of the value of sympathy and engaged dialogue.

But the survey did not find that doctors investigate the patient's mind as a correlative of what is actually happening in his or her body. I am certain that the great majority of doctors realize that prolonged unhappiness or stress makes one "susceptible" to a host of ailments. Yet they disregard this "first cause" of disease and focus their attention on the "final cause"—the virus or bacteria, the arrhythmic heartbeat, or the arthritic neck.

Even psychiatrists, whose entire practice involves healing the mind, only recently have defined psychosomatic illness in terms of a clear mind-body link. "Psychosomatic" no longer denotes an illness that exists only in the imagination, but one that moves from the imagination to the body. Stomach ulcer was one of the first diseases acknowledged to be caused by a mental state—not by certain foods or by a stomach dysfunction.[106] The psyche (mind) affects the soma (body) and causes not imagined stomach pains, but real perforations in the stomach lining. Other diseases linked early on to state of mind were spastic colon and high blood pressure. Today, probably due to the influence of Hans Selye's groundbreaking research on stress, most diseases—from the common cold to cancer—are believed to be stress-related. And what is stress but a state of mind?

Selye proved not only that stress weakens the body's defenses, but that the enemy was not "out there" but "in here": Individuals possess different stress thresholds and also react differently to such common stressors as loss of employment, marriage, divorce, relocation, the birth of a child, and so forth. It is the way a situation is perceived, not the situation per se, that either precipitates or deflects illness.

Selye's conclusion has been confirmed in a multitude of studies. One study, which investigated the incidence of streptococcal infections among 100 people in 16 families over the period of a year, found no association between streptococcal infections and (1) the number of streptococci present, (2) the allergic history of the patient, (3) the presence or absence of tonsils, (4) changes in the weather, (5) type of housing, or (6) family size. It did find a "strong and remarkable" association between streptococcal as well as other respiratory infections and acute personal family stress.[107] Viruses and bacteria can make little headway if an organism is not already weakened by stress.

The correlation between stress and breast cancer is so startling—women who have been unhappy for a period of years have a 50 percent greater incidence of cancer—one wonders how the medical profession can approach prevention in any other way. The big headlines and the big funding goes to researching the 5 to 10 percent of breast cancers that supposedly are linked to DNA. The mental connection is virtually ignored.

In my own case, I haven't the slightest doubt that the disease was psychosomatic—a perfect example of Selye's theory that ongoing stress coupled with repressed rage causes adrenal exhaustion, which in turn is tied to any number of maladies. I know now that my unhappiness for the two years preceding the diagnosis inevitably would cause an illness of some kind. Why cancer of the breast, why not of the spleen or the colon? Why cancer at all? Why not MS or a heart attack? I had no hereditary background for any of these. The nature of my unhappiness selected breast cancer from the whole array of possible maladies as the disease most symbolic of my internal disease. My psyche chose the one disease that perfectly demonstrated the feelings of unworthiness and shame that had troubled my spirit from the time I was a child. When I reached puberty, what I regarded as underdeveloped breasts became the anatomical evidence of this unworthiness. My breasts were the locus of my shame in the geography of my psyche. That is the way illness works: Illness is a physical signpost of psychic disorder. If we are prepared to look, illness points us to the root problem.

A disease feels as though it has fallen upon us from the outside. But the first cause lies within us. Our moods and emotions and ideas—internal events—cause something to happen externally. The external event is then blamed for the presence of the mood, emotion, or idea. This circle of cause and effect is probably what Charles Fillmore, cofounder of Unity, meant when he talked about consciousness "trapped in its own effects."

The trickle of concession from mainstream medical practitioners that the mind affects disease is recent and, compared to 20 years ago, sizable. Still, many die-hard doctors adamantly refuse to appreciate the mind's role in the condition of the physical body. Because of their high status in medical circles, I chose Dr. Marcia Angell, editor-in-chief of the *New England Journal of Medicine*, and Dr. Barrie Callileth, of the University of Pennsylvania Cancer Center, to represent the stance of the die-hards. Their remarks reveal the stubborn resistance of the entrenched medical model: "Medical literature," says Dr. Angell, "contains very few scientifically sound studies of the relation, if there is one, between mental state and disease." And again, "It is time to acknowledge that our belief in disease as a direct reflection of mental state is largely folklore."[108]

Dr. Callileth agrees: "We do know that it [the effect of mind and emotion on illness] is not a direct cause-and-effect relationship." Dr. Callileth warns against "the increasing numbers of practitioners around the country who offer mind tricks as cures for cancer."[109] And Dr. Angell worries about making patients feel guilty by suggesting to them that their minds may affect their disease: "If the power of positive thinking doesn't work and the cancer spreads, the patient is burdened with guilt by having to accept responsibility for the outcome," she laments. One implication of that remark is that if chemotherapy doesn't work, the patient will feel better because he or she can blame the doctor.

Of course Dr. Angell misses the point. Taking responsibility is not the same as feeling guilty: Taking responsibility is a recognition of one's free will—not just concerning the past and illness, but concerning the future and health. It is a sad commentary on our social and religious mores that they too often force us to feel guilty about the actions and thoughts we take responsibility for. There is either innocence: "I had nothing to do with it," or guilt: "It is my fault." Guilt stems from helplessness. Guilt and self-blame are themselves disease-inducing states of mind—they themselves have to be shed for healing to take place. We recognize the role of our own minds, not to castigate ourselves, but to enlighten and empower ourselves. Taking responsibility allows for searching for a better way.

While relatively few doctors acknowledge that a distressed mind contributes to sickness, and even fewer see that a well mind contributes to health. Practically none—not even holistic doctors—factor in the soul. Soul is not a *reality* in the practice of medicine. Only a handful of now famous and extraordinary doctors such as Bernie Siegel, Larry Dossey, and Herbert Benson, and the psychologist Lawrence LeShan see the possibility of curing the body through the mind and soul.

Bernie Siegel caused a great stir with his book *Love, Medicine, and Miracles*. Since its publication in 1986, he has been one of the most sought-after speakers in the country—traveling to universities, talk shows, and medical conferences. His message, startling at the time, is that love is therapeutic and that the spirit is indeed connected to the spleen in a direct—if not instantaneous —cause-and-effect relationship.

Likewise, Larry Dossey urges the importance of examining the life values of the patient as part of the treatment. He advises doctors to "look at meaning as seriously as we look at the cholesterol level or the blood pressure."[110] He points to studies conducted by institutions with mainstream credentials like Johns Hopkins that have come up with conclusions as striking as these: (1) The greatest predictors of cardiac problems and low-back pain are not heredity or body type or general health, but job satisfaction and general happiness. (2) The greatest risk factors for cancer are poor love relations with parents during childhood and the inability to express emotions. (3) Fifteen minutes of meditation twice a day lowers cholesterol.

In Dossey's view, the mind, the psyche, and the spirit contain healing powers only dreamed of in most medical theory. He asserts that unhappiness and lack of love cause illness, and that meditation stimulates health, and he is unequivocal in his claim that prayer has the power to heal. He cites studies that prove that not only the patient's own prayers, but also the prayers of others, aid the healing process—even when the patient is not aware he is being prayed for.[111]

Norman Cousins, a magazine editor, not a doctor, in his book *Anatomy of an Illness*, probably did more than anyone to validate holistic medicine. By abandoning conventional treatment, he recovered from a connective tissue disease for which the prognosis was total paralysis. Obeying his intuition, he checked himself out of the hospital with its invasive, rest-disturbing routines, subnutritional food, and destructive medications—all of which he felt were worsening his condition every day—and took himself to a comfortable hotel room where he not only recovered but did so at one-third the cost. The treatment he invented for himself combined massive doses of vitamin C and laughter: vitamin C for his collagen, laughter for his mind and emotions. A few weeks later, he got out of bed and returned to his desk as editor of the *Saturday Review of Literature*.

Here at last was an important voice that not only testified to the benefits of holistic medicine but reached beyond holistic medicine to the ultimate power of the mind. With trenchant insight, Cousins speculates that both the vitamins and the laughter that healed him were placebos: "There is a possibility of the affirming emotions enhancing body chemistry." Even more pointedly, he says, "Creativity, will to live, hope, faith, and love have biochemical significance." He mentions especially and repeatedly the curative power of a "robust will to live."

Disappointingly, toward the end of the book, Cousins recants his own assertions and experience. Driven by motives difficult to fathom, he pulls the rug out from under his own feet by warning the reader not to take what he has stated too seriously. One should not succumb, he says, to "irresponsible disregard of genuine symptoms." And again, "There are times when medication is absolutely essential." Does this mean that his own symptoms were not "genuine," or that before he abandoned the hospital, his physician did not prescribe medications that were felt to be "absolutely essential?"

Also unfortunate is Cousins's refusal to support the American Holistic Medicine Association. He gives two reasons: (1) its antagonism to mainstream doctors and (2) its indiscriminate mingling of such acceptable remedies as acupuncture with such exotic practices as astrology. If Cousins took his own statements on the placebo effect seriously, why debunk astrology or anything else that leads the mind to have faith in health?

Except for a scant handful, like LeShan and others mentioned in chapter 17, "Breakthrough Medicine," even those doctors who stand on the threshold of admitting the mind's power back off from crossing a forbidden line. Most books that advocate a departure from conventional medicine contain caveats similar to Cousins's: "If you are experiencing a serious health crisis, I urge you to consult your personal physician." "Faith, expectation, and suggestion may produce miracle cures, but [a cure for] terminal cancer is a bit too much to expect."[112]

Lawrence E. Jerome, the author of *Crystal Power: The Ultimate Placebo Effect*, for example, after proclaiming for a hundred pages the power of the placebo, ends with a disclaimer that undercuts the crucial point of his book: "Unfortunately, no amount of faith, crystal-power, hypnosis, placebos, or alpha training can cure the physically deaf, or the two blind men. . . . [They] can help only in certain ailments: pain, and conditions controllable by the human mind."[113]

If Cousins and the doctors I have mentioned, advanced as they are, had stood by their convictions, if they had declared that nothing—neither an outside organism nor a malfunction of the physical system—can cause illness unless it first takes hold of the mind, I would be writing this book only as a testament to their truth. But all of them retreat from their fundamental insights. One can only wonder why: Is the truth too large to encompass? Do they fear lawsuits, or slander by the medical or scientific communities? Do their publishers insist on modifying their message? Are they reluctant to propose a path to people who are not ready to walk on it?

Who knows? I can only surmise. Perhaps "holistic" doctors are afraid to trust their own portentous words, for then they would be forced in all good conscience to abandon medicine as they now practice it. Essential to their continued practice is the conclusion that while illness may be mediated by the mind—that is, reduced or intensified by it—the mind neither creates nor cures it. I myself took 13 years before the truth was established so deeply in my consciousness that I could proclaim it without a qualm.

⁓

The unwillingness of these farsighted doctors to stay out on the limb they've risked going out on may relate less to medical conviction than to philosophy. Our culture is philosophically committed to dualism— mind is one thing and matter is another. If this is so, it becomes necessary to solve the puzzle, of how mind can cause something to happen in matter: how mind can leap over the chasm, so to speak, that separates it from matter. In practical terms, how can a thought cut a hole in your stomach?

Holistic medicine, like conventional medicine, conceives of the human being as a duality, a mind and a body—two distinct aspects, albeit stitched or woven together. Some holistic medicine, adding a soul to this equation, conceives of the human being as tripartite—a mind, a body, and a soul, each requiring the care of a distinct specialist—a physician for one, a psychologist for the other, a priest for the third.

I believe that we won't be able to utilize the full power of the mind until we realize that these divisions are fabrications. We don't need holistic medicine to be integrated into conventional medicine—we need *monistic* medicine. Monistic medicine would operate on the premise that the body is not reached *through* the mind or *through* the emotions, but that a human being is composed of *one substance* of which body, mind, and soul are simply three modes of demonstration, just as water, ice, and vapor are three modes of demonstrating H_2O, and waves and particles are two modes of demonstrating light.

The metaphysical riddle of how the mind, a nonmaterial thing, can affect the body, a material thing, vanishes if body and mind are the same thing—different modes of being, not different kinds of being. The mind is matter or else the body is mind; if not, intercausality could not exist.

～

How could we explain the heightened effectiveness of a drug when it is administered by an empathetic doctor except to conclude that the doctor's manner instills confidence in the patient? A good bedside manner is a placebo. Prayer is a placebo. The laying on of hands is a placebo. If a placebo, a mere nothing, can produce an observable outcome, aren't we forced to admit that the curative agent is not external to the patient, but, rather, is the patient? In the language of the Bible: "The Father within doeth the work."

I believe that the medicine of the future will concentrate on triggering placebo effects. Encouraging patients to have faith in their ability to cure themselves will produce more cures than are dreamed of in our present medical philosophy. Doctors will be doctors of the spirit.

"What about science?" you ask. This *is* science. It is the science that science has not yet caught up with.

15

countless cases of nonmedical cures

If there has ever been a case of tuberculosis healed spiritually, then germs are not the cause of tuberculosis.
— Joel Goldsmith

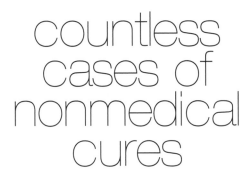

Shouldn't we be alarmed when a doctor suffers from the disease he treats others for? "Physician heal thyself" is a completely justifiable request. We have every right to ask, "How can you presume to help me if you cannot help yourself? Let your own good health give me confidence in your method."

I would not have the temerity to speak to you about self-healing if it had not taken place in my own body. I would not point you toward a path I had not traveled. Many have gone farther than I; sharing their experiences would be a great service to all of us.[114]

Until the writing of this book, my story was known only to friends and relatives. There are legions like me who don't write books and whose experiences therefore are known only in their immediate circles. The general public becomes aware of nonmedical healing only when the person is already famous or becomes so—Mary Baker Eddy, for example, or Myrtle Fillmore, both of whom experienced healings that led to the founding of new religions.

But if the general public were to purposely seek out accounts of "miraculous" healing, their findings would fill volumes. Occasionally we hear by word of mouth about someone's astonishing recovery from a terminal disease. Or we read an occasional newspaper or magazine story about a health "miracle." But these tales are too rare to warrant serious interest; their rarity removes them from everyday life. They influence our ideas about health in about the same way that Halley's Comet influences our ideas about the night sky. If we heard every day about the nonmedical cures that occur every day, we would be more inclined to believe they were possible, and that belief, in itself, would make them occur more frequently.

Unfortunately, there is practically no place to look for current cases of nonmedical healing besides the weekly *Christian Science Monitor* and the monthly *Christian Science Sentinel*. Between 1971 and 1981, these papers published over 4,000 case histories. Because

Christian Scientists do not differentiate illness of body from illness of mind—an intestinal problem, say, from friendlessness—most of the cases relate to conditions such as poverty, loneliness, job failure, and family tragedies. Christian Scientists believe these ills of the spirit come from the same place as bodily ailments and are cured in the same way. The 4,000 cited cases do include 1,430 cases of purely physical maladies of widely diverse kinds. Of these, 655 had been medically diagnosed and recorded. All of these patients refused medical treatment, but all of them returned to a doctor for a follow-up examination. The medical follow-up found that of the 655 problems, 655 had disappeared.

The case of Ellen Hendel, who lived in Dorpat, Estonia, illustrates a Christian Science mental process. At the time she learned she had tuberculosis, she was not a Christian Scientist. She had heard of Christian Science but had dismissed it. After trying all conventional treatments, as a last straw she decided to visit a Christian Science practitioner.

She writes: "Five and a half years ago I was a broken-down individual. . . . According to physicians, I was suffering from tuberculosis; and they gave me only a short time to live. . . . I was surrounded at that time by dark impenetrable night, as it seemed to me, and death was awaiting me. As nothing was known about Christian Science at that time in Dorpat, I went to Riga, where I immediately received loving treatment from a Christian Science practitioner. After three treatments the cough left me, and after eight I was healed. This healing took place quite suddenly. I was walking along the street when it

became *tangibly* clear to me that I as God's perfect like-
ness, must reflect health, and that I lived, moved and
had my being in Him; and all at *once it seemed as if something fell from me*, I felt so light and happy—and I knew
and felt that I was well. . . . There is no language in the
world with which I could express what I felt at that time.
I could, in my overflowing joy, have exclaimed to everybody, 'Rejoice with me, for I am well!'"[115]

Mormon literature, especially of earlier times, also
contains many accounts of nonmedical healing: "Elsa
Johnson had had a rheumatic arm for many years, and
for two years had not been able to raise her hand to her
head. . . . The prophet walked up to Elsa and said,
'Woman, in the name of the Lord Jesus Christ I command thee to be whole,' and then he walked out of the
room. Mrs. Johnson was instantly healed and the next
day she did her washing without difficulty or pain."[116]

Mormon lore also tells of a "massive" charismatic
healing. At a Mormon settlement in Commerce, Illinois
(later known as Nauvoo), an outbreak of a malaria epidemic in July 1839 felled almost the entire congregation.
The prophet Joseph was also deathly ill but, "when the
power of God rested upon him" he left his bed and went
out to administer to the congregation: "He did not miss
a single house, wagon, or tent in the entire compound
and then along the bank of the river. He walked into the
cabin of Brother Brigham Young, who was lying very
sick, and commanded him in the name of the Lord Jesus
Christ to arise and be made whole. He arose from his
sick bed healed." Together they healed everyone in the

congregation.[117]

Records of other healings tied to religious beliefs come from the Emmanuel Church. The Emmanuel Movement was founded in the late nineteenth century specifically as a healing ministry. It based its practices on biblical evidence that people can be healed through a combination of prayer and the power of suggestion. The success of the Emmanuel Movement became legendary. Here is just one report from a practitioner: "I could cite examples which might seem extravagant or of doubtful truth, but, leaving those aside, I may relate one instance of recent occurrence: A prominent man of about sixty was lying very ill in a private hospital. His physicians did not seem hopeful of his recovery. [He suffered from] perforations of the lungs resulting from asthma, complicated by gas inhaled during the war. . . . When his family first asked my cooperation the physicians demurred on the ground that his condition was a purely physical one and not amenable to psychic or spiritual treatment."

However, the patient was rapidly losing ground; and as the physician felt there was nothing to lose, he allowed the Emmanuel practitioner to visit. The practitioner (who was able to visit only once a week because the patient was in another city) writes, "For some little time he showed no sign of improvement save the relief of better sleep." One day the practitioner was informed there would be no use in going in, as the patient was unconscious and apparently near to death. But the practitioner implored permission to minister to him as usual, and was permitted to sit at his bedside where the practitioner carried out his usual treatment of prayer combined with autosuggestion, used to induce the patient's faith in his own healing. A remarkable recovery occurred soon afterward: "the lesions and perforations in the patient's lungs healed with such rapidity that six weeks later he was fishing for tarpon."[118]

Religious literature being the foremost repository of nonmedical cures does not help spread the word and may actually undermine acceptance of its validity: Members of one religion tend to doubt miracles when they occur in the religion of another; and of course, non-religious people reject the idea of miracles entirely. That is why understanding the placebo effect is so important. Everyone—atheists, agnostics, and people in all belief systems—can agree that it occurs. The placebo effect proves that healing is available to anyone who can awaken a deep faith in a cure—any cure.

If reports of nonmedical cures were disseminated by the scientific community, both religious and nonreligious people might give them more credence. A recovery seems less like a miracle when the testimony comes from a doctor, say, a heart specialist like Dr. Brugh Joy, or a psychiatrist. One psychiatrist who had begun to meditate writes: "It was remarkable. My whole life changed. First, I noticed that I was healing myself. I used to regularly sprain my ankle playing tennis. Almost every month I would be laid up for a week with a swollen ankle." One day, after another spraining episode, she went upstairs to meditate, and when she came down, realized that she bounded down the stairs: "The swelling in the ankle had gone down and it wasn't sore. I was totally amazed."[119] As a result of this experience, she continued to study meditation and visualization techniques, and began to use them on her patients, whose afflictions ranged from sexual problems to cancer.

For his part, Dr. Joy—who received his medical training at the prestigious Johns Hopkins Medical School—actually left the practice of medicine after he had experienced a nonmedical healing. In his important book, *Joy's Way*, he tells the story of his recovery from acute pancreatitis. During the time he was afflicted with the disease, he searched his mind for a psychological explanation of his terrible illness: "Why was I manifesting a disease process that could severely restrict my activities or take me out of this plane all together? With each attack I explored the circumstances that surrounded it, trying to find some pattern. I examined the stresses in my life but they were inconsequential in comparison to the disease and thus not powerful enough to lead it. I talked to my body, trying to find some symbolic aspect that a malfunctioning pancreas might reflect." The vocabulary Dr. Joy uses—"manifesting," "symbolic aspect"— indicates that he already saw the connection between mind and health, but his disease was still active.

One day, during a meditation, a "call" came to change his life. The call was to trust completely in the power of the spirit—not only for the healing of his body, but also for the healing of his life. He gave up both his medical practice and his academic teaching position. He gave up his car, house, and furniture, and embarked on a journey that included Findhorn in Scotland and the pyramids of Egypt.

Since the day of that meditation, he has not had a

single attack. Finally, he founded Sky Hi Ranch—where the goal is for patients to heal their bodies by healing their spirits.[120]

The French writer Honoré de Balzac relates that as he walked through the streets of Paris he frequently "absorbed" the personalities of passersby "through his skin." Something of the same sort of ESP often occurs in the realm of nonmedical healing. Dr. Joy's healing began with a mysterious "knowing" or deep intuition of conditions not discoverable by the senses or by instruments. The Emmanuel Movement practitioner Edward Worcester says that sometimes he has intuitive knowledge of the cause of a patient's suffering, and when that happens, he knows he will be able to help him.[121]

Probably the most widely known ESP health practitioner in America is the late Edgar Cayce. Many of his diagnoses and treatments (including that of his own illness) came to him in dreams. Usually he entered a trance state and began the diagnosis with the words, "Yes, we see the body." He left records of 30,000 cases, typified by an account of a woman who came to him crippled by arthritis and abandoned as incurable by doctors: Cayce put her on a regime of exercise, massage, and a special diet—which had come to him while he was in a state of trance. She followed his instructions and was cured.

Another case of trance diagnosis in which Cayce correctly "saw" a spinal disorder—overturning a doctor's previous diagnosis of appendicitis—made the *New York*

Times. This case was particularly important because the patient himself was an MD, Wesley Ketchum, who had wrongly diagnosed his own ailment. The publicity made Cayce famous and brought the sick flocking to his door.[122]

I have mentioned that Mary Baker Eddy was unremittingly maligned by the medical community. Edgar Cayce, far less antagonistic to conventional medicine than Eddy, was virtually hounded. Unlike Eddy, he did not forego material remedies or withdraw from the world of the senses. In fact, he worked in tandem with an osteopath, and often arranged for his patients to be treated by physicians. He welcomed new technologies; and receiving instructions while in trances, he himself invented several therapeutic electrical and magnetic devices. Even so, his success did not inspire medical research; instead, it stiffened opposition. In 1945 he died poor and worn out by the unrelenting antagonism of the medical organization.

I must add that the vigilance of the conventional medical establishment in protecting its turf continues. The February 5, 2001 issue of the *New Yorker* tells the story of Dr. Nicholas Gonzalez, an MD who received his credentials from Cornell University, which is affiliated with the Memorial Sloan-Kettering Cancer Center. Gonzalez had become deeply impressed with the work of Dr. William Donald Kelley, an orthodontist, who was widely recognized as an authority on nontoxic cancer treatment. Like Kelley, Gonzalez adopted a cancer treatment approach that strengthened the immune system and cleansed the body of toxins. To do so, he tailored a dietary/nutritional regimen for each patient—an approach much like the one practiced by the doctor I briefly turned to in 1982 (chapter 1). Kelley had been denounced by the American Cancer Society, and now Gonzalez came under even more severe attack: The New York State Medical Board rebuked him for "departing from accepted practice," and he was required to take psychological tests and to undergo retraining.

But like Mrs. Eddy and Mr. Cayce, Gonzales stands his ground: "There is really only one truth," he says. "Either cancer patients get better with my treatment or they do not. And, if they do, I could care less whether it involved moon dust or microbes from Pluto. . . . And what has that made me in the eyes of the traditional cancer establishment? Simple. I am Gonzalez, the quack, the fraud, the doctor who lies to cancer patients, steals their money, and kills them."

I mention Dr. Gonzalez primarily to reveal how impossible it is for any unorthodox treatment to escape attack. As to the efficacy of Dr. Gonzalez's treatment, I base it on the attitude of his patients. As one of them says, "You hear something horrible is going to happen to you and you have to put your faith in something. . . . And this is where I put it."

Everyone is unique, but everyone who has been healed has something in common—they *believed* they would be healed. In every case, something or someone caused the individual to trust that he or she would be healed—a gesture, a word, a ritual, an environment—or a doctor, a priest, a hypnotist, a spiritual teacher. On the other hand, healing fails when, no matter how patients strive to have faith that something will cure them, they *really* believe they will remain sick or die.

~

The medical model of disease, especially the current medical model of cancer, evokes such terrible fear that only an extraordinary patient could decline the drastic modes of treatment authorized by medical convention and instead summon the faith in healing that their recovery requires. Dr. Robert P. Heaney's friend succumbed, as most people do, to convention. Dr. Heaney tells his story in the article, "What Choice Did He Have?"[123]

"I lost a good friend the other day. He died, some might have said, of cancer. But that is not accurate. He died, actually, of surgery, of medical intervention—of medical hubris, really. He did have cancer, an early one, discovered incidentally in the course of evaluating a largely unrelated complaint. The surgery was directed at the cancer, of course. It was a technically difficult and chancy procedure—well performed, so far as one can tell—but of a sort that the human body does not tolerate well and often does not tolerate at all. In any event, my friend's body did not; after four trips to the operating room and nearly 20 hours under the knife, he died. He had entered the hospital three weeks earlier, ostensibly a well man."

Dr. Heaney continues to say, "What is this technological tyranny in which so many of us so willingly collude? In what other sector of our lives do first-world

citizens experience such total capitulation, such uncondi-
tional surrender, as to the medical surgical forces arrayed
against cancer? It is capitulation not to the enemy itself,
but to the tyranny of forces that we hope may save us
from that enemy. It is as if citizens of a democracy gave
up their freedom and submitted to a dictatorship in
order to ward off an external assault on that very freedom. Can we not see that the cure may sometimes be
worse than the disease?"

And I say, coming from where I have come: How
unfortunate that Dr. Heaney's friend had "early detection." How unfortunate that he, with the encouragement
of organized medicine, felt terror so strong that he acted
precipitously and wrongly to exorcise what he had been
told was the "enemy" from his body.

Timothy Ferris says in *The Mind's Sky*, "If we were
to meet a higher order of being who knows how to affect
the physical world using methods we do not possess,
we would discount it as magic." All of the people mentioned above, patient and healer alike, have affected the
physical world using methods we in fact do possess. If
these people are a higher order of being, they are not
higher because they possess unusual abilities but because
they have *the will to believe* these abilities.

16

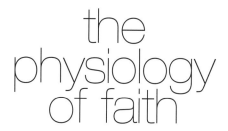
the
physiology
of faith

Awareness produces chemistry.
—*Deepak Chopra*

I have said that my religious revelation brought with it an instantaneous change in my relationship with life. Before then, life had seemed sometimes vibrant and plentiful, sometimes deflated and empty—an amalgam of the good and the bad, the beautiful and the ugly. My revelation transformed the world: Now it was ineffably beautiful, unalterably perfect, and inescapably eternal—as, I realized, was I myself. It never entered my mind to wonder whether something in my brain chemistry, in the grey matter within my skull, accompanied my moments of transport.

Since then I've learned that science supplies proof that brain functions do change when thoughts and feelings change. But proof has come with exasperating slowness, and its impact on the general practice of medicine has been almost nil.[124] It still is the medical fringe group that researches and expounds the fact that intangible psychic functions affect physical brain functions.

For myself, I don't need to know exactly what physiological processes accompanied my revelation. I don't need to name endocrine fluids or brain chemicals, just as I don't need to analyze the composition of the sun in order to grow flowers; I only need to realize that flowers thrive in a sunny spot. Yet I wouldn't doubt that my ecstatic state produced a flood of whatever electrical and chemical outputs of brain and gland help cure the body.

I wouldn't doubt that physiological changes occurred, but I insist that mind and spirit caused them. The medical model reverses the sequence of these events: It fully grants that endorphins bring a feeling of well-being, that a physical substance can cause a state of mind, that being healthy can cause you to be happy. But it is wary of and unwilling to grant the opposite: that feelings of happiness and well-being precede and are the source of such chemicals as endorphins. The medical model admits the proposition that being cured can cause you to have faith. But it declines the proposition that having faith can cause you to be cured. (You'll recall Dr. Callileth's insistence that cancer cannot be cured by "mind tricks.")

If a placebo has cured even one person, it seems to me the placebo effect should be the primary target of medical research.

Despite the relative lack of research, the idea that the mind has the power to heal is so potent a truth that it has infiltrated even traditional medical specialties. One immunologist, noting that sufferers of Chronic Fatigue Syndrome usually have pretty high antibody levels, treats the disorder as an immune system problem, yet includes psychotherapy in the treatment. She explains, "The immune system is very much affected by mood states. Depression definitely causes suppression of T-cells." And "love," she says, "really does heal. . . . Being in love is really being in love within oneself, and that has a positive effect on the immune system."[125]

That the immune system seems to affect all healing from a paper cut to cancer is an idea creeping into the minds of even the most backward physicians. None but the most advanced, however, asks what affects the immune system. Doctors know, for example, that there is a link between allergies and the immune system, yet they don't seem to be concerned with the link between the immune system and the mind. The accepted explanation of allergic reactions says that the body attacks an innocent substance, which it mistakes for a destructive invader. Dr. Dan Kinderlehrer, co-author of *Food Allergies*, goes much further. He maintains that the mistaken attack is in some sense "permitted" by the mind, and his approach to allergy treatment pays careful attention to the many levels at which human beings function: biochemical, cellular, organic, psychodynamic, and spiritual.[126]

Early scientific investigation of the way the mind affects the body concentrated on degrees and thresholds of pain. One study investigated the amount of pain dental patients experienced when their teeth were extracted without anesthetic. As expected, the pain was great. When a placebo was given, the pain was ameliorated or completely eliminated. The *unexpected* finding, the serendipity, was that placebo mimicked a "real" painkiller in more ways than one. Researchers were astonished to find that when a drug that *blocks the action* of a "real" painkiller (the opiate antagonist naloxone) was given, it blocked the painkilling action of both the real drug *and* the placebo. In other words, when the patient was given a placebo, he felt no pain; when he was given a placebo plus a drug that interferes with the action of painkillers, he again felt pain.

This experiment clearly points to three conclusions, the import of which has yet to penetrate conventional medicine: First, the patient's expectation controls his experience; put another way, *faith* in the treatment *is* the treatment. Second, when a placebo produces a beneficial result, the benefit can be negated in exactly the same way the benefit of a "real" drug can be negated; put another way, loss of faith in the treatment thwarts the treatment. This experiment did not measure endorphin release, but in the light of studies that have followed, a third conclusion can be offered: The dental patients' state of mind—either the expectation of relief or the expectation of an obstacle to relief—triggered or failed to trigger the production of opiate-like chemicals, endorphins, in the brain. To put that another way, a spiritual state (faith) produces a material substance (brain chemicals).

Endorphins, immunity, allergies, and pain—the list of proven physiological effects from states of mind doesn't stop there:

Documented studies show that (1) stress affects blood glucose levels in diabetics and (2) blood sugar levels of diabetics have been lowered by placebos. Both of these would be impossible unless some sort of psychological mechanism were involved in the production of blood sugar.[127] Yet the usual doctor treats blood sugar malfunction as if it were determined by genes and exacerbated by diet.

Most doctors do recognize the connection between the adrenal gland and emotions. Great fear causes the blood pressure to fall—sometimes dramatically enough to cause death. In fact, adrenaline surge might be the scientific explanation of death from hexes; the hexed person is literally scared to death. Adrenaline surge is involved in a whole variety of psychophysiological phenomena—the "fight or flight" response, panic attacks, and the ability to lift heavy weights or run at extraordinary speeds. Here we have proof that a secretion from a gland can save you or kill you.

The medical approach to this phenomenon stops at the gland. The mental approach goes back to the state of mind that triggered the gland. The adrenal gland is merely the factory that produces a chemical according to instruction from a nonphysical force—the idea that there is something to be afraid of.

Research has proven that anger, like fear, causes toxic substances to be manufactured by the body. The course of events goes something like this: An angry person produces toxins that pour into the bloodstream. In order to regain its balance, the body produces antitoxins. Thus the body poisons itself and then becomes exhausted trying to rid itself of these self-induced poisons. If this dynamic occurs frequently, the person suffers—among other undesirable outcomes—adrenal exhaustion and becomes ill. Research on these phenomena concentrates on the body's endocrine system, and the treatment of endocrine imbalances is performed on the body. Because fear and anger are mental phenomena, it seems to me that the logical treatment for adrenal exhaustion would be psychological or psychospiritual. But only a handful of MDs, with Deepak Chopra at the forefront, acknowledge the primacy of the mind in the endocrine system.

Scientific experiments often "discover" what we have always known. One such experiment came to the conclusion that nervousness causes some kind of "action" to take place between the nervous system and the salivary, pituitary, thyroid, and endocrine glands. This action is "involuntary, automatic and sub-conscious."[128] My question is: If the experiment had not arrived at that conclusion, would it have convinced us that nervousness does not make the mouth dry and the armpits wet? That fear cannot release a trickle of urine or tenderness a trickle of tears? The sad answer to that question is yes. Science can talk us out of the evidence of our own senses.

The significance of the toxins-anger relationship is as relevant to the health of society as it is to the health of the individual. Repeatedly we hear that the principal cause of the high percentage of illness among poor minority groups is the lack of medical attention or nutritious food, whereas the primary cause may be incessant anger. Even factoring in lifestyle excesses such as multiple sexual partners, drugs, and violence, the much higher rates of illness and mortality among ghettoized minorities can be due to the unremitting stress caused by actual and perceived prejudice. Continuous hostility coming from, or believed to be coming from, the dominant group must arouse anger in the "victim" group, and anger experienced either consciously or unconsciously may cause toxins to pour continually into the bloodstream.

After reviewing a broad body of evidence, psychiatrist Robert Hahn postulates exactly that: Independent of other risk factors—for example, smoking, alcoholism, and high-fat diet—"a person's position in the larger society significantly affects his or her morbidity and mortality." One study he cites found that the blood pressure of migrants is lower before than after they migrate, and that migrants who lived among people of the same origin had a smaller incidence of heart disease than those who live with the members of the "new society." In other words, the psychological impact of minority status is, in and of itself, deleterious to health.[129]

Despite overt and covert pressure to conform to conventional medical practices, new fields of medicine have emerged: Neuroimmunology and psychophysiology and, more recently, psychobiology and cyberphysiology, take seriously the implications of the placebo effect. Says one psychophysiologist: "As investigators have come to learn more about psychosomatic medicine and about psychological and social determinants of disease, they

have attempted to develop a comprehensive psychophysiological theory capable of explaining the placebo
effect."[130]

Fields of inquiry removed from the practice of medicine per se support the basic concepts of psychophysiology and cyberphysiology.

Wilhelm Reich, Ida Rolf, Alexander Lowen, Moshe
Feldenkrais, Irmgard Bartenief, among the most famous
of bodywork therapists, consider states of the body as
clues to states of mind. Instead of approaching the body
through the psyche, they approach the psyche through
the body. Whereas traditional psychotherapists correct
physical problems—for example, impotence, migraine
headaches, and colitis—by balancing the psyche, bodywork therapists correct psychological disturbances by
balancing and harmonizing the body.

And, as mentioned earlier, Kirlian photography—a
process that photographs the energy (heat) surrounding
objects—has verified the claims made by mystics and
psychics that each of us is surrounded by an aura, the
colors of which reflect our emotional and physiological
"temperament." These auras are found universally in religious tradition. Holiness is marked with a penumbra of
radiance or by unnatural brightness of the countenance.
The Hebrews who witnessed Moses' descent from Mount
Sinai said that his face radiated light. Jesus, Mary, and
the saints are depicted with golden or white auras
around their heads. A halo orbits the Buddha's head.
Some people say they can see auras with the naked eye
and can interpret the state of mind and health of the

subject by the hues, size, and shape of the aura. I am told that a relaxed and happy person emits a larger, brighter, and differently colored aura than does a tense or depressed person.

I stated earlier that we know we have reached the boundary between knowledge and ignorance when we face a paradox. Studies of "the interaction between the nervous system and the immune system . . . have produced conflicting results. . . . [Yet there is] overwhelming though mostly anecdotal clinical literature supporting a much larger influence."[131] What can be going on if the empirical evidence of the laboratory only scantily supports the "overwhelming" empirical evidence of experience?

What is going on illustrates the limitations of the scientific method. The scientific method seeks to prove something by manipulating a limited number of "relevant" variables. But if one takes a holistic view of human beings and their place in the wholeness of their environments, then all variables are relevant, and they are infinite in number. The scientific method can learn only about that which it can hold under the microscope and only for as long as it can hold it there. Once the boundaries of the sample are expanded, either temporally or spatially, everything changes. Cancer cells in the body of an individual behave differently than cancer cells in a test tube or cancer cells in the body of another individual.

No doubt the science of the future will be able to

"prove" that a patient's expectations and his personal and cultural symbols affect his health, in just the same way it has proven that fear causes an adrenalin surge, without however, probing more deeply into the physiological significance of expectation and symbols. Expectations and symbols are metaphysical influences; science cannot prove them "real," for each individual response to a symbol is unique. Widespread anecdotal evidence is more, not less, trustworthy than laboratory proof because when the phenomenon under observation in the laboratory appears in real life, it appears in the flux of real life, amidst an infinitude of uncontrolled variables. Science does not invent reality, it adapts it to its own lexicon, which is partial and slanted to support its own methodology. Whatever science "finds" was already there, like an America before Columbus discovered it.

If I expand the microscope metaphor to include every instrument from the telescope to the periscope, the metaphor still captures the limitation of the scientific vision: Dealing with the material world, it can develop and test hypotheses only on material forms. Beyond this, its conclusions are no less "imaginary" than the visions of a religious mystic.

Placebo effects are the bane of conventional medicine because they stand as proof that people heal themselves, and that is a proposition medicine can hardly accept and remain medicine as it is currently practiced. When, in the future, medicine recognizes that the mind reigns over every physiological event, it will no doubt invent medical terminology to explain effects that have no external cause.

Dr. Howard Brody, author of *Placebos and the Philosophy of Medicine*, says, "As we learn more about specific physiologic and psychologic mechanisms of drugs and other treatments, the realm of effects now attributed to placebos will shrink."[132] The realm of effects attributed to placebos might shrink, but only because as science admits the enormity of the number of placebo effects, it will give these effects more medically acceptable names. The placebo effect may be called "non-inductive cerebral response phenomena," but it still will be a cure caused by nothing but the mind of the patient.

Every religion, one way or another, associates physical health with spiritual health. Every philosopher has had to engage the question of how the nonmaterial world affects the material world—a question dealt with briefly in chapter 14, and one that must enter any discussion about the physiology of faith. If the spirit is a different order of reality than the body, how can the spirit affect the body? The unique way science answers this question forms the underpinning of biomedicine and accounts for the kind of gross discrepancies between the laboratory and life that puzzled Dr. Howard Brody.

The practice of medicine is always tied to a definition of the human body, and that definition in turn is tied to a definition of what is real. Both definitions have changed over time. In ancient times in the West, the body was first seen in terms of outer form and structure—weight, height, musculature, complexion—

to which temperament was somehow related. Later, the internal body entered the picture and temperament was associated with various bodily fluids—the humours. Quite recently, the cellular level was discovered, and after that the molecular level and DNA. Most recently have come the submolecular, atomic, and subatomic levels. These complete the present definition of the material body. But the last two of these do not suggest a solid material body at all. Instead of material, we find swirls of energy fields interactively undulating. Between these energy fields, and far larger than the energy fields them- selves, we find huge spaces—nothingness. The human body and every variety of matter is made up mostly of nothing. Conventional medicine, as it is now practiced, cannot incorporate these implications of modern physics.

Some years ago Russian scientists conducted an experiment in which petri dishes containing yeast were placed in front of one group of people whose eyes were open and another group whose eyes were closed. The yeast grew significantly more when it was being looked at. The scientists concluded that "the eyes of the observer emit a force field that can influence what the eyes are looking at"[133] and, additionally, that this energy is meas- urable and of a different intensity in different people.

The "connector" between the object and the subject in the yeast experiment is called a force field, also called the astral dimension (Theosophy), the Magnetism that binds all things to all things (Paracelsus), and *prana* (Hinduism). In modern times, before Einstein, this connector was called ether. All these terms suggest mysticism or, to a scientist, the downright foolishness of ancient error.

A recent breakthrough book by the Cambridge University biologist Rupert Sheldrake, *The Presence of the Past*, posits the idea of morphogenetic fields, a dimension of reality composed of fields that contain and preserve nonmaterial events—the ideas, thoughts, and emotions of all times.[134] This "storehouse of memory" would account for such phenomena as ESP and the collective unconscious (Jung). It would also account for the hundredth-monkey phenomenon—the observation that ideas are "contagious" and that when an idea is present in a certain critical number of minds, it is mysteriously transmitted to virtually everyone, spreading through the air, so to speak, like an epidemic.

When you think deeply about the possibility of self-healing, you find yourself propelled into larger philosophical questions about the nature of reality. The province of medicine is the material world. Individual doctors may be deeply religious—but *in their role as physicians* their concern is the physical, not the metaphysical. Indeed, some religious doctors may find the bifurcation of their world very troubling. When a patient comes to them with an illness, the illness is perceived as residing in their material beings, and the treatment—drugs, surgery, or what have you—is performed on their material being.

Belief systems can be divided into four categories based on their theories of mind/matter: dualism, materialism, idealism, and monism. Dualists, those who believe that matter and mind both are real and diametrically opposite, are immediately faced with a tantalizing conundrum concerning the action of one upon the other. How does emotion, a thing of the mind, penetrate flesh? How can one's feeling become one's physiology? How does an abstraction like love cause a concrete thing like a heart to flutter and the blood to be concentrated into a blush? How does a nonmateriality like fright cause the automatic peristaltic action of digestion to be reversed into vomiting? To answer that the feeling of love impels some kind of endocrine action or releases endorphins in the brain, or that fright causes a flow of adrenaline, begs the question: It describes the result; it doesn't explain how thought can leap the gap between mind and matter, how a mental hammer can pound a real nail. New fields like neuroimmunology have clearly proven that a cause-and-effect relationship does exist between mind and matter, but it has not answered the "how" question that is posed by dualism.

Materialists avoid the entire dilemma. Matter only, in its various forms, is real. The metaphysical—mind or spirit—is an epiphenomenon, a delusion, or a kind of hallucination created by naming something that isn't there. Matter acts upon matter, brain chemicals work upon the material nervous system; there is no mystery to be solved regarding immaterial cause and material effect: The physical hammer drives the physical nail.

Materialists cite brain surgery and strokes to prove that there is no mind independent of brain—when a part of the brain is lost, a part of the mind vanishes. "Thinking is a biochemical event," says mainstream psychiatrist Aaron Beck. And even George Dawson, author of

Healing: Pagan and Christian, says that "mental events are in some way dependent upon certain brain events." Experiments on healthy brains seem to substantiate these materialist views: A brain will produce a thought or a feeling when an electrode is implanted in a selected brain site; the electrode prod causes the brain to reproduce a past experience or stimulates a specific memory trace.

But do strokes and brain probes really prove that the mind is the same as the brain? Not at all. For one thing, many areas of the brain are "silent" and have yielded *nothing* to experimental probing. What goes on in those areas? For another thing, the response of the brain to a probe in no way tells us what the brain responds to when there is no mechanical or electrical probe. What "probes" the material brain to produce a memory or a feeling? What stimulates ideas and emotions? If materialists answer that sights, sounds, odors, tastes—in other words, the senses—transfer impressions from physical objects to the physical brain, they would have to postulate some sort of material conductor in the space between the object and the nervous system.

But even this would not prove that the locus of thoughts is the material brain. A myriad of thoughts can accompany any single sense impression. If the sight of a dandelion causes a poet to think, "the body of a green girl/stands en pointe/balancing her being's gold," can the flower be responsible for the thought? Neurons might fire and chemicals flow, but they do not create metaphors and symbols. Teilhard de Chardin said, "To think we must eat, but what a variety of thoughts we get out of one slice of bread." If, as materialists may contend, the chemicals and electrical circuits of the brain are the brain's way of continuously probing itself, the brain would be hermetic; how would a new thought break in? The brain continues to be a mystery to science because science is fundamentally materialistic and cannot acknowledge that mind is different from brain.

Unlike materialists, dualists do not regard the brain as the source of thoughts, but rather as a kind of storage trough of thoughts—in the same way that a tapestry stores the weaver's thoughts or a recipe stores the thoughts of a cook.

Idealists (or those who believe only spirit is real), are materialists' polar opposite, allowing only the metaphysical realm of existence. They say that mind is not a product of matter (brain), but rather that brain is an invention of mind. "Matter" is the naming of something that isn't there—a delusion, an error of belief. Mind affects mind, spirit affects spirit, and neither affects matter, because matter is only a shadow on the wall of a cave.

Christian Scientists are the pragmatic idealists of our time. They *practice* the nonexistence of matter as a tenet of faith, and consequently reject medical treatment. In *Science and Health with a Key to the Scriptures*, Mary Baker Eddy says, "The opposite of Truth,—called error, sin, sickness, disease, death,—is the false testimony of false material sense, of mind in matter. . . . Christian Science reveals incontrovertibly that Mind is All-in all, that the only realities are the divine Mind and idea. This great fact is not, however, seen to be supported by sensible evidence, until its divine Principle is demonstrated by healing the sick. . . ." If idealists are correct, however, then we are speaking with non-mouths, causing non-sound waves, writing on non-paper about a non-health issue, and the least absurd non-course of non-action would be to remain silent.

Unqualified idealism drops us into a welter of pointless and unnecessary problems. To deny material reality—the flutter, the blush, the adrenal surge, for example—is as groundless as the materialist's denial that there is such a thing as mind that causes these reactions. When, as research has proven, the brain has been triggered to produce the chemical prostaglandin by thought alone, materialists deny that thought is the cause and idealists deny that the effect is prostoglandin.

There is a fourth solution, the only one that seems reasonable to me:[135] Matter and mind are the same thing. Reality is monistic. In religious terms, God is One. Mind and brain are different manifestations of the same substance, different wavelengths, so to speak, of one energy. Monism has been ridiculed as an example of *reductio ad absurdum*, a reductionism that responds to all questions with the same answer. Reductionism has an unsavory reputation; to accuse a scientific or philosophical theory of being reductive is a way to invalidate it.

Reductionism also lends itself to comedy: A boy in one of Kurt Vonnegut's stories, having been told that God is everything, looks wonderingly at his little sister drinking a glass of milk—here is God (milk) contained in God (cup) being drunk by God (girl). A disputant may well ask, "When you say that the composition of everything is identical—all is all—what have you explained?"

Nevertheless this is what monists do say, and it is what quantum physicists also say. Monism is the philosophy that underpins the healing of the body by the mind.

The fact that psychic states affect the ductless glands was discovered 60 years ago. At that time, Dr. Elwood Worchester stated that "beyond question our mental and moral condition affects these glands."[136] Yet it has taken 60 years for doctors like Bernie Siegel and Herbert Benson to incorporate this idea into actual practice.

More than 80 years ago, in 1910, a Dr. Williams, writing in the *British Medical Journal,* tells of chorea being provoked by fright, an attack of gout being caused by a fit of anger, and an exophthalmic goiter brought on by worry and anxiety.[137] Dr. Williams doesn't temporize his belief: "Serious disease," he says, "may be caused by morbidly dwelling upon the idea that one is suffering from or will suffer from some dreaded illness. Such persistent direction of attention . . . sometimes produces the feared effect. . . . Contrariwise, a resolute confidence that a cure would be vouchsafed has accomplished that end."[138]

It has taken more than 80 years for these ideas to take hold—and only of relatively few physicians. The great majority warn, as even a forward-looking doctor like Oscar Janiger warns, that "ascribing a moral or spiritual subtext to an illness can be dangerous. . . . Beliefs must be tempered with hard facts and common sense. . . . If taken to an extreme, patients might forgo effective treatment."[139]

I don't want to end this chapter on that negative

note. In the 1930s, several researchers took EEG equipment to India to study certain physiological processes of enlightened individuals. They did indeed find that these enlightened individuals, yogis, could control their physiological processes and achieve a state measurably different from that of most people.[140]

One leading physiologist, R. Keith Wallace, informed the Twenty-Sixth International Congress of the Physiological Sciences that the EEGs of enlightened people revealed a state different from either a sleep state or a waking state: a hypometabolic state that he described as a state of "restful alertness" (a state Dr. Benson more recently renamed "the Relaxation Response"). These findings became the rudiments of biofeedback training, and the state of restful alertness is known to neurologists as alpha, a state that carries a sense of inner peace. Biofeedback training has been accepted into conventional medicine, but although doctors use it therapeutically, they don't use it to prove the truth that mind governs matter.

Recently an astounding connection was found between traumatized children and the biological processes in the bodies and brains of these children as adults. Dr. Bruce Perry, psychiatrist and neurobiologist affiliated with the Baylor College of Medicine, found that years after the traumatic events, "the effects of abuse, neglect and domestic and community violence show up in heart rates that alternately race and plummet. . . . The child's *body* is damaged by what he *witnesses!*" Dr. Frank Putnam, chief of the unit on developmental traumatology at the National Institute of Mental Health, clearly sees the import of this mental phenomenon: "The idea that [stress and trauma] truly impacts physiology and biology . . . is a very scary thought."[141]

You cannot be healed by any method you do not have faith in, and faith cannot be forced upon you. But faith, or lack thereof, is contagious. We have "caught" faith in medical cures. Very few doctors take note of the prodigious number of nonmedical cures. And those few certainly do not credit faith for these cures. The idea that *all* physiology begins in the mind and that nothing but the mind is necessary to accomplish healing has been accepted by a minority too small to call tiny—a lunatic fringe to some, way-showers, to me. A few of these doctors appear in the next chapter, "Breakthrough Medicine."

17

breakthrough medicine

Healing takes place when you claim it.
— *Evander Hollyfield*

I hope the preceding chapter made clear that this book is not about the value of emotional support for the sick. It is not about helping the patient achieve a better frame of mind in order to facilitate conventional medicine. It is not about humanizing doctors and their procedures—the day of the god-doctor and unquestioned faith in medicine has already been diminished by the inroads of alternative and holistic medicine. This book is about the power of every individual to cure himself or herself. It is about the realization that if the mind is powerful enough to assist medicine, as holistic doctors assert, it is powerful enough to dispense with medicine, as practically nobody asserts.

It is all too easy to disregard anomalies such as people who live healthfully on and on despite prognoses of imminent death or people who are cured by faith healing. Anomalies are unimportant annoyances until so large a number accumulates that they demand to be explained. "Faced with such phenomena," says doctor Oscar Janiger, "one kind of physician will shrug them off, attributing them to spontaneous remission, placebo, coincidence, or the power of suggestion, as if these labels should settle all further inquiries."[142]

One wonders how it is possible to shrug off evidence that the power of suggestion has cured tuberculosis or crippling arthritis, or to pay no attention to an "anomalous" case like the following, having to do with the mind's ability to control pain:

The patient had been obtaining some alleviation of chronic pain through the use of cortisone given by her doctor. She consulted with a second doctor who explains: "I felt the temporary relief of cortisone was not worth the side effects of long term use, like joint degeneration. I got to know this patient. She liked and respected me, and she knew I was trying to help her. I would tell her I was giving her an injection of cortisone, but I was actually using a placebo. . . . A little belt of saline solution in her buttock gave her three or four days of relief, just as if it had been cortisone."[143]

Far more amazing examples of the mind's control of the body appear in medical archives, both past and present:

Peter Parker, an American surgeon and missionary, reports that back in 1843 he performed a mastectomy on a Chinese woman who, after the operation, "raised herself up from the table without assistance, jumped upon the floor and made a bow to the gentlemen present . . . and walked into the other room as though nothing had happened."

Another surgeon, named J.F. Mitchell, in the early 1900s performed amputations, thyroidectomies, and other major surgery without general anesthesia. More recently, Theodore Kocher, a Nobel laureate, reports that he performed 1,600 goiter operations without general anesthesia.[144] A firsthand account comes from a dentist, Dr. Victor Rausch, who had used hypnosis on his patients and wanted to verify the outcomes on his own body: In 1978 he had his gallbladder removed without anesthetic or painkillers. He was awake throughout the operation and left the operating room on foot. Rausch reports the hostile reaction of a surgeon who hadn't performed the surgery: He "looked at me, stuck his finger in my face and said 'I don't want to hear about it. I don't want to talk about it.' For him to accept what just happened, he'd have to discard 90 percent of what he had learned."[145]

"Breakthrough" doctors are doctors who have begun to see that anomalies are the rule.

On the surface, breakthrough doctors resemble holistic/integrative doctors. The difference is that holistic doctors see psychological and spiritual elements as supplements to basically orthodox practices, while breakthrough doctors see orthodox practices as the supplement. When a convinced breakthrough doctor employs conventional therapy, it is primarily as a concession to patients who cannot trust too radical a departure from the norm.

There must be a greater number of breakthrough doctors than my research has turned up, yet they are few enough to be considered the renegades of medicine, suspected by their colleagues and rejected by agencies that finance research grants.

I closed the preceding chapter, "The Physiology of Faith," with reference to the state of restful alertness that can be learned through biofeedback training or achieved through meditation. Breakthrough doctor Karen Olness trains her patients in biofeedback and other self-regulation processes. Olness is a professor of pediatrics, family medicine, and international health at Case Western Reserve University's School of Medicine, as well as the director of international child health at Rainbow Babies' and Children's Hospital in Cleveland, Ohio. Her credentials, by conventional standards, are impeccable; but her practice of cyberphysiology is neither conventional nor, in the estimation of National Institutes of Health, impeccable. NIH has never awarded her a grant in a breakthrough area despite her successes.

Under her care, children have overcome excruciating attacks of migraine headache, debilitating attacks of asthma, and unusual susceptibility to infections. She uses no medications and employs no invasive procedures. She uses self-hypnosis, applied biofeedback, autosuggestion, visualization, and other methods of self-regulation. She judges her procedures successful only when the problem has been completely eliminated, and she is successful in 80 percent of the cases.

In 1987, Olness published a study in *Pediatrics* that should have catalyzed the entire profession but that inspired only a couple of young MDs to follow her lead. Her study proved that self-hypnosis could elevate levels of salivary Immunoglobulin A (IgA): Children trained by Dr. Olness became less susceptible to disease, using only the self-induced belief that they *could* elevate their IgA.

Approaching a child's illness through the child's mind, she has cured maladies found intractable by conventional medicine. In fact she is usually the "referral of last resort," as in the case of Bess:

Eight-year-old Bess was afflicted, as her mother and her aunt before her, with migraine headaches that incapacitated her with blinding pain for hours at a time several times a week. Before her referral to Dr. Olness, various doctors had treated little Bess for four years with a variety of medications—including the drug of choice, Propranolol—with no success. Olness eliminated the drug; and on her first visit, she coached Bess in a biofeedback technique for lowering galvanic skin response (GSR) by shrinking an image on a computer screen. When the image shrank to nothing, Bess had attained a state of complete relaxation.

On the second visit, Bess achieved the same state by allowing Dr. Olness's voice to guide her: "Every time you breathe out, enjoy relaxing . . . all the way down to your toes." When fully relaxed, Bess was invited to imagine "a place where you like where you are, and you like how you feel." Then, Dr. Olness put Bess in charge of her own physiological functions by asking her to imagine a switch or a button—any device of her own choosing—that was able to turn off pain. "You're the boss of that control," the doctor assured her, and continued guiding her deeply into what I have defined as a state of faith—faith in her own ability to rid herself of pain. During the two weeks following the second session, Bess had only one headache, an improvement unmatched in the preceding four years.[146]

This child was the beneficiary of Olness's earlier study that showed that cyberphysiological treatment of migraine in children is more effective than Propranolol. Olness's more recent study of mind over matter trained nursing mothers to use techniques of mental self-regulation to increase IgA in the mothers' milk. Think of the benefits to humanity if women could be routinely trained to increase the IgA of breast milk—here would be a simple, self-empowering, and cost-free way of increasing the nourishment of infants.

I have mentioned Dr. Bernie Siegel and Dr. Larry Dossey—both serious holistic practitioners. Dossey emphasizes the healing power of prayer, and Siegel emphasizes the healing power of love. Neither fits into the category I am calling "breakthrough" because neither maintains that the mind is the sole—or even the princpal —source of healing. Nor has a third, famous holistic doctor, Deepak Chopra, fully substituted mind for medicine. Chopra (an endocrinologist), like Siegel and Dossey, has gone far beyond most doctors in asserting the importance of the mind, but, like them, he has not gone all the way in clinical practice. His ideas about mental healing, as presented in his best-selling books, derive from the spiritual traditions of India. He writes, "Medicine is trying to understand health by studying disease. The whole strategy is wrong, and based on the superstition of materialism which says that matter is primary and consciousness is secondary." And again, "The fact is that our perception is what is creating our reality, even on a molecular level." His statements perfectly encapsulate self-healing theory, but he has not done what Karen Olness has done—he has not treated patients through the mind alone.

Dr. Lawrence LeShan, a research psychologist, comes close to asserting unequivocally that an individual can heal himself. LeShan began his research into faith healing as a skeptic, but not a closed-minded skeptic. He was suspicious of the claims of faith healers, but he wasn't content to repudiate them without investigating the evidence that such healing occurs. He determined to test the verity of faith healing by training himself to be a faith healer. He studied accounts of faith healing and found that two features appear in all of them: (1) Faith healers perform some kind of ceremonial activity—such as ritual bathing, lighting candles, prolonged seclusion, or prolonged prayer—in connection with the healing session. (2) At a certain point, the healer undergoes an alteration of consciousness, a shift away from the world of common sense.

Because most religions advocate, and religious mystics engage in, meditation, LeShan adopted meditation as his training discipline and entered an intensely demanding regimen: He meditated six to eight hours a day, five days a week. For a year and a half, he practiced several different meditation techniques and, always the scientist, kept notes on each.

At the end of a year and a half, while still a skeptic, he had his first result as a healer and, he says, it "scared the living hell out of me." He was working with a woman whose arthritis had prevented her from closing her fingers into a fist for over a year. During her session with LeShan, she merely sat and read the newspaper while he attempted to achieve in himself a state of altered consciousness. For two or three fleeting seconds, he achieved such a state—he felt his and the woman's identities become one. According to LeShan, the woman had no idea what was going on, but she left the session having recovered 59 percent of mobility in her hands.[147]

LeShan first overturned his own skepticism by accomplishing a faith healing. Later he realized that it is not he who is responsible for the healing, but rather that he promotes healing by inducing a state of faith. A faith healer inspires faith; the healer is the patient.

Breakthrough medicine empowers the patient. It does what psychotherapy is supposed to do—it leads the patient out of a habitual mindset into an awakened state of consciousness. Psychotherapists expect changes in mind to produce changes in behavior. (Some psychotherapy specialties, e.g., health psychology, expect changes in body function, as well.) Breakthrough doctors expect changes in consciousness to produce changes in health.

We begin to see that breakthrough medicine may not be "medicine" at all, as we now understand it: It may be more like group prayer or religious affirmations or Silva Mind Control or EST (currently The Landmark Forum). Did Dr. Olness practice medicine on Bess? Her technique probably bears less resemblance to anything she learned in medical school than to Transcendental Meditation. Maharishi Mahesh Yogi, the famous originator of TM, has commissioned numerous scientific studies, that show that TM produces a state of restful alertness—exactly the state Bess achieved under the guidance of Dr. Olness. Maharishi also says, "One of the most important elements in practicing the TM technique correctly is an innocent, non-analytical attitude." Perhaps Olness's success is due in part to the innocence and youth of her patients: They haven't yet developed fixed ideas promoted by biomedicine—which most adults need the force of a calamity to break through.

I have no doubt that breakthrough medicine is the medicine of the future, though doctors will arrive there via different paths. You can hear the medicine of the future breaking through in the psychologist P.D. Borkovec's comments on the placebo effect: "For me the placebo effect represents one of those amazing 'realities' that on my pessimistic side indicates how little we know about human behavior . . . and on my optimistic side hints at what incredible potential may exist within human psychological abilities. The possibility that what one believes to be true may actually influence what does become true is nothing short of spectacular in its implications."[148]

Doctors may be propelled toward a new medicine by dint of their own successful experiments or by the force of their own insights. In his book *The Evolution of Modern Medicine*, Dr. Oscar Janiger has collected a slew of statements from doctors who seem to stand on the brink of practicing breakthrough medicine.

One physician began to study metaphysical phenomena and found that they led her to recast her role in the processes of her patients' healing: "As physicians we can simply act as catalysts for the expression of that healing spirit within us. . . . The liberation of one's spiritual forces can optimize healing, and I looked for methods that would not countermand the wisdom of the body by suppressing it with allopathic drugs or surgery."[149]

Another physician who prays for his patients and sometimes with them, tells about an elderly man with tic douloureux—a malady characterized by facial pain so excruciating that it can depress the sufferer to the point of suicide. The afflicted man had seen a number of specialists and was considering neurosurgery. The doctor stated: "When I saw how his emotional situation was deteriorating, I volunteered that we should pray about it. We did, and he broke down and tearfully said that he had never shared a prayer with a physician before.

Over the weeks and months after that, he said the pain was gradually going away. We stopped talking about neurosurgery and decreased the medication to almost nothing." The cure, or near cure, this doctor believes, combined divine intervention and the patient's faith that such intervention can occur: "He was able to make use of his conviction . . . that God was hearing his prayer and easing his pain."[150]

Still another physician, a surgeon, operated on a

woman who'd had 23 of 26 lymph nodes test positive for cancer. Cancer had appeared at the base of the tongue—a variety of cancer with a survival prognosis of 0 to 5 percent. Yet she has been in remission for 18 years and leads prayer and faith healing groups in her home.[151]

One obstetrician sounds like an Edgar Cayce with medical credentials (see chapter 15). He explains that since early teenage years he had psychic powers, and, as a doctor, he is able to "see your body from head to your toes." He "knew" that one of his patients had liver problems the moment he walked in. "I talk to people's bodies, kinesthetically and telepathically. I might ask the liver how it's doing, and I get an answer, either a feeling or a vision. I work a lot with women who can't get pregnant. One woman in her late thirties hadn't been able to become pregnant for three or four years and was traumatized by all the drugs she had to take. I asked the spirit of the child who wanted to enter her body why it couldn't. The spirit replied, 'Because her pituitary isn't strong enough.' She appeared healthy but I gave her pituitary supplements and herbs. She got pregnant."

Reflecting on such experiences, the doctor says, "You know, there's a part of me that is astounded by all of this. Yet, I can also feel very matter-of-fact about it and say, 'I don't think this is crazy at all.'"[152]

Most doctors would think this was crazy—even those who have witnessed "apparently unaccountable recoveries from serious illness," such as the recovery from terminal cancer of a patient of a brilliant London surgeon. The surgeon had operated three times on a man who had cancer in the lip, which had spread to the glands in the neck. The surgeon refused to perform a fourth operation. But the mass began to decrease in size and finally sloughed away. Five years later, the man was perfectly healthy. "Perhaps it is scarcely true to say that the body has these powers," writes George Dawson, author of *Healing: Pagan and Christian*, reflecting on this case: "It seems rather to be a matter for the entire personality, which impresses itself upon the bodily powers and is able to induce reactions which destroy conditions inimical to life. The recovery is natural and not supernatural."[153]

After such knowledge, it is difficult to understand why a physician would continue the practice of conventional medicine. I'm baffled. But a few doctors at least are listening to voices that lie outside the Hermes box of orthodoxy.

Science deals with laws of matter. Spiritual science deals with laws that transcend matter. Breakthrough medicine is medicine that has broken through from matter to the science of mind. If you believe in the laws of matter as the only or primary laws, then the principles that govern matter will govern your life and the power of the spiritual will recede from your life. If you believe that the laws of spirit are primary, then the laws of matter will recede.

If we are to usher in the new age of breakthrough medicine, we must get over our notion that the products of science are facts and the products of mind insubstantial nothings. Scientists themselves often point out that science is a human contrivance. The assignment science has taken upon itself—to objectively examine objective phenomena—is technically impossible. All phenomena are filtered through three lenses: the human mind, the singular mind of an individual scientist, and the approaches that are peculiar to the scientific method. C.P. Snow speaks of the findings of science as an "edifice," a piece of architecture that is a "wonderful collective work of the mind of man."

If breakthrough medicine is a practice that uses the mind to heal the body,[154] then doctors of psychology and psychiatry, more than medical doctors, would be its most obvious practitioners. Certain schools of psychology do stress the power of conscious mind: Cognitive therapy and Rational Emotive therapy claim that the power of destructive events can be defused by altering the way patients describe these events to themselves. Gestalt therapy claims that the external world of the patient can be changed by teaching the patient to focus on the here and now—the time and place where the mind and the body are one—instead of on the past or the future. Logotherapy claims that patients can achieve fulfillment by realizing that the events of their lives have significance beyond themselves—that is, that each person can create a transpersonal vision of his or her own life.[155] And the great Italian psychologist Roberto Assagioli, in an approach called Psychosynthesis, practiced creative visualization long before conscious imaging was called by that name. Assagioli taught, in effect, that if his patients could hold in mind a different way of being, that way of being would come to pass in their lives.

Whether psychological concepts like these filtered into New Thought religions or the other way around, cross-fertilization has certainly occurred and impacted breakthrough medicine. Creative visualization, for example, which is nothing more—or less—than mental pictures or fantasies the mind creates to "persuade" the body to alter its condition, is a mainstay of Theosophy, Unity, and most other metaphysical or "science" religions. It is also the approach that distinguishes the famous Simonton Clinic in Texas: At Simonton, children may be told to picture in their minds a bunch of good guys driving off the cancer-cell bad guys. They then reinforce this mental image by drawing a picture of it on paper.[156]

Before his breakthrough, Dr. Brugh Joy was a cardiologist using conventional procedures to treat heart disease. When his own grave illness was cured by nonmedical means, he left the practice of medicine and founded a health ranch where metaphysical healing is employed. He sees the role of the doctor completely differently from the one taught in medical schools. He says, "No matter what physicians do, they can only augment the healing process of the body itself. . . . The human mind can and does generate force fields that can transmute matter."[157]

Dr. Joy has formulated a healing process that engages only the mind. In his book *Joy's Way*, he outlines the six steps his patients are instructed to follow:

1. Relax as completely as possible. All tension must be released. If during the relaxation some part of the body begins to tense, pay attention. Identifying areas difficult to relax will help you see where you carry most of the tension in your

body, and this understanding may lead to deeper psychological insights.

2. Recapture the memory of an inspirational experience. Live it again. This trains the emotional and feeling areas of consciousness to flood the body with a sense of well-being.

3. As you image the happy memory, allow all the good feelings you felt at the time to flood the body now.

4. Know that this feeling and state of consciousness support the healing process. Direct the flood of good feelings to the problem area. Feel it wash through. Trust that it is going to every cell in the problem area.

5. Visualize the problem (disease) actually improving, becoming less and less, and finally being replaced by pleasure. Don't worry about how this is being done. The body knows how to heal. Your work is to see and feel the problem disappearing, and to see and feel the healing energy filling in.

6. Visualize yourself being perfectly well. Feel the well-being of perfect happiness.

The Emmanuel Church, Transcendental Meditation, and Alcoholics Anonymous (AA) offer closer models of the medicine of the future than does today's orthodox medicine. The Emmanuel method cures through prayer and autosuggestion; TM leads to peace of mind that encompasses peace of body; and AA appeals only to the mind and spirit, yet has cured more cirrhosis than liver specialists, more unemployment than employment counselors, and more broken families than psychotherapy.

But these practitioners and organizations are few, and the strongest of them, AA, thinks of itself as a road to spiritual, not physical, health. AA spawned the most widely used group therapy concept of our time—the Twelve-Step program—which has been applied to everything from managing companies to incest survival. But while Twelve-Step programs abound for coping with all manner of nonmedical problems, no program as yet uses the Twelve-Step concept to cure medical problems. Such a development would be an excellent means of bringing self-healing to thousands.

In every field, practical application trails far behind theory, and common sense trails far behind practical application. Medicine seems peculiarly prone to a time lag. Antecedents to breakthrough medicine can be traced to the early eighteenth century, when a priest, (with the embarrassing name) Dr. Hell, collaborated with Franz Mesmer on a theory of celestial bodies' influence on the minds and bodies of humans. He also postulated a subtle, mobile fluid that pervades the universe, unites everything, and affects the nervous system. In the meantime, Mesmer presented in his doctoral dissertation the idea of "animal magnetism"—the effect, intentional or unintentional, of one mind upon another. Mesmer and the priest parted company when Mesmer repudiated the influence of the planets and began, with great success, to heal people by manual contact and passing his hands in slow movements before their eyes. As we saw previously, he practiced an early version of hypnotism.

Later, Chevalier de Barbain, a student of Puyseg (who was a student of Mesmer), practiced suggestion in a form that today we would call guided meditation or affirmation. De Barbain would sit by the bedside of his patients and instruct them to repeat after him certain words and to think healing thoughts. In 1813, the French naturalist Deleuze published *Histoire Critique du Magnetisme Animal*, stating unequivocally that "faith is essential in order to obtain any cure."[158] And we have already seen how Mesmer influenced Phineaus Parkhurst Quimby, how Quimby influenced Mary Baker Eddy, and how Eddy both reflected and influenced New Thought.

Now, almost 200 years later, mental theory is being taken seriously in medicine—but only yet in medicine's most marginal fringe.

In chapter 16, "The Physiology of Faith," I mentioned a study on the painkilling potential of placebos, which concluded that placebos can cause the release of morphine-like substances in the nervous system. Unexpectedly it was also found that naloxone, a drug that interferes with the effects of morphine, also interfered with the morphine-like action of the placebo. Simply put, a placebo exactly imitates the effects the patient expects from the active drug. Another double-blind study raised doubts about the validity of double-blind studies themselves, for it was found that the doctors affected their patients' reactions: The doctors in group A were aware that they were giving two kinds of injections, a placebo and Fentanyl. The doctors in group

B also were aware that they were giving two kinds of injections, a placebo and naloxone. The patients in group A experienced relief of pain whether they were given the placebo or the drug. The patients in group B experienced an increase of pain whether they had received the placebo or the drug. Apparently, the doctor's expectation of a certain result was itself a placebo effect that outweighed other placebo effects.[159] It is frightening to think how much the course of a disease may be influenced by the doctor's attitude toward it.

We may never know all the ramifications of Dr. Olness's success. Is it her faith in the treatment? Is it her suggestion to the patient? Is it the autosuggestion of the patient's self-induced hypnotism? All of the above? We do know what her treatment is not—it is not a drug.

Neither Dr. Olness nor little Bess *willed* the cessation of migraine headaches. The doctor eased Bess into improvement; Bess *surrendered* to healing. We don't choose health—or anything else—with our will; we choose with our whole being. The will is analogous to post-hypnotic suggestion—it doesn't lead, it follows what the mind has already chosen.

In our society, we admire brains and will power. But it isn't really our brains or our will that drive us. It is our heart and our unconscious. A man's will might say, "I want to meet a nice woman." But he spots just the wrong woman across a crowded room and is attracted to her. In exactly the same way, a sick person says, "I want to be well." But his unconscious mind says, "I *am* sick! I *am* sick!" "I am" is far more powerful than "I want." "I am" encompasses one's total identity. "I want" implicitly means: The thing I want is beyond me; I do not yet have it and I am worried that I may never have it. "I want" expresses a belief in something missing: I *want* health because I *am* sick. In this state of consciousness, the person remains sick. As we'll see in the next chapter, the will is less powerful than the imagination.

18

fighting disease —a losing battle

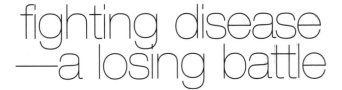

In a contest between imagination and will,
imagination will always win.

—*William James*

I have often been asked why, after eight years, I
decided to have a lumpectomy. The answer is simple: A
few months before the surgery, I began to fear the lump.
I don't know why, but I do know that the unconscious
mind turns fears into causes—fear, in and of itself,
initiates disease; if my fear remained, the lump would
have to be removed.

But for eight years the lump and I were on good
terms; I felt a kind of friendship toward it, as one might
feel toward a spider that has taken up residence in
the corner of the room. At times I regarded it almost

affectionately. I patted it—it was faintly visible to the naked eye and easily discernible to the touch—and I was willing to allow it to be part of me, provided it didn't overstep its bounds. I even talked to it: "Little lump, everything has a role in God's scheme of things, so there must be a reason you're still here." Or, at times when I was in a magnanimous mood: "Who is to say my life is more valuable than yours? Let's agree to live compatibly. Just stay where and as you are. Don't attempt to take more *lebensraum*, and we can live in peace together."

I believed then, and since then my belief has been strengthened and validated, that everything in our lives serves a purpose—not excepting that lump in my breast. We call forth events and conditions because we need them: They serve us in one way or another, and the lump served me in many ways—some I understood at the time, some I have gained insight into over the years.

First of all, the lump prevented me from thinking that what had taken place was a miracle. If the physical sign of cancer had disappeared at the time of my mystical revelation, I would have been tempted to believe God had intervened. Instead, the lump exhorted me to consider other possibilities about the relationship between God, myself, and my health.

It also kept me humble. After the revelation (during which I kept asking, Why me?) I felt specially chosen; I was God's avatar; I was a new Jesus. Was I supposed to fast for 40 days? Climb a mountain? Proclaim to the world that I had seen God? "Don't be so proud," the lump admonished me, "many have seen God."

And it questioned my readiness to speak to the

world: It warned me that before I thoroughly understood my healing, my story might do more harm than good. It advised me to wait for the right time and the right way to deliver the good news that we hold our own health in our own hands.

The waiting was not easy. God had given me an assignment but had not given instruction for fulfilling it. I often felt guilty and helpless; I was supposed to do something, but what? The lump's presence sometimes frightened me into holding my tongue, other times dared me to have the courage to speak out in spite of its presence. I tried to console myself with John Milton's famous words, "He also serves who only stands and waits." I reminded myself that we never know the effects of our actions—what may seem like an insignificant act of kindness, a stray word, a feeling of love toward someone or some thing may reverberate to the good of the universe more forcefully than what appears to be grand and notable. So while I "stood and waited," I tried to practice these small acts, and I found that making my life a small model of the good was far more difficult than writing this book.

But now, as I write this book, I am sure the lump had to be there for another reason. Had it disappeared there would be no way to "prove" I had cancer. The typical reaction of most people would have been skepticism; either my imagination or my veracity would have been suspect. The original biopsy report would be attributed to error—a misreading of the results or a mix-up of my breast tissue with another's. Had the lump vanished, no second doctor, eight years later, would have confirmed the diagnosis. In short, I needed the lump, which is another way of saying I wanted it: It supplied me with irrefutable material evidence upon which to base the message of this book.

I take it as an infallible principle that life delivers to you what you want. Having said that, I admit that sometimes it is not easy to figure out what you want; what you really want hides under layers of "the right thing" to want. That hiding from our subconscious desires is, of course, the whole basis of psychoanalysis.

But what you really want sends strong signals from underground. The signals take the form of discrepancies between what you think you want and what you get: You claim to want health yet are sick, to crave love yet are lonely, to attain economic comfort yet are poor. A professed desire for health often veils a buried desire for illness. To illustrate, let's say you have a cold. "Darn this cold!" you complain. Now you can't deliver the speech you've been working on for a month! Or, now you can't take that long-awaited vacation. Or, now you can't spend the night with that special person. You'll swear, of course, that you really regret not being able to do these things, and you would probably become angry with any amateur psychologist who suggested that the cold—annoying as it is—delivers very real compensations: While you are on vacation, your competitor might move into your job slot; the special person is pressing for a commitment you're not ready to make; the very thought of the speech makes your stomach turn over.

Those benefits lie near the surface of conscious mind. The benefits may be more sly:

1. As a child you had frequent colds; you have always been "somebody who gets colds," colds are part of your identity. Not getting colds would somehow require further changes in your identity.

2. Everybody gets colds; there's a kind of cold-catcher club. If you didn't get colds, you would be out of step and deprived of the commiseration that goes with "belonging."

3. You *believe* in germs. They are out there and people who bump into cold germs get colds. People who believe that one's state of mind brings on colds are kooks, so you'll just "catch" this cold from someone who sneezed in your vicinity to prove that you are not responsible. Where colds —or any other illness—are concerned, you are a hapless victim.

4. Your husband and your children have colds. It would be very thoughtless of you, cold-hearted even, to remain in robust good health while your loved ones are sniffling and sneezing away. It would be like feasting while they go hungry. (Plus you'd be expected to nurse all of them.)

5. It's unreasonable to expect to be perpetually healthy. Life isn't like that. And besides, illness is a kind of chastisement; you certainly have done things you deserve to be punished for.

These examples of possible hidden benefits are my own inventions. But the underlying principle is the same for all of us. Search your own mind and you will discover that beneath the apparent distress of the cold (or any other negative circumstance in your life) lies something you want. If you are willing to face this unpleasant possibility, you can set yourself on the path to well-being.

Before 1982, I would not have dared to say what I am about to say—the unconscious "benefit" of illness might be death. I have never heard of anyone who had a potentially mortal illness saying they did not want to live. If pain is severe they may wish to die, but only because death presents a way of escaping pain or of ending the terrible deterioration of the body. If a cure were possible, they would want to live, or so they say. Haven't they fought to live? Haven't they undergone the unbearable tortures of treatment? Who would dare to suggest that perhaps getting the disease in the first place was a way to escape from living?

"A person can make herself sick, and that same person has to will herself to get well again," says Beverly in Carol Shield's novel, *The Stone Diaries*. But "will" is a tricky word; willing is an ambiguous faculty of the mind. Sometimes it means merely to wish or want or desire. Sometimes it means wish, want, or desire stiffened by the intention to bring something about. And sometimes intention translates into action; but when it does, I maintain that something different than willpower in the usual sense was involved.

Despite the oft-repeated belief that people who get well possess a strong will to live—a "robust" will to live, as Norman Cousins phrased it—the *will* to health is not the way to health. The way to health is *submission* to health. It is will in a peculiar sense: You will yourself to *give up* illness; you will yourself to *let* health overcome you. Dr. Larry Dossey writes eloquently about the power of doing nothing and the power of denial, and that is exactly what I mean: The "action" of your will is, in a sense, a nonaction. You quit the struggle. You do not fight the disease; you release it.

The word "denial" has a very negative connotation in our culture. No one wants to be accused of "being in denial"—the posture of an ostrich or a coward. The negative meaning of the term "denial" is appropriate for some situations, of course: We think of the woman who blinds herself to her husband's obvious escapades, or the drunk who refuses to admit his alcohol problem. On the other hand, unfortunately, "denial" is too often the label attached to optimism and faith. A person who refuses to accept a bad prognosis is said to be "in denial." But is that so? Refusing to succumb to bad news, taking responsibility for your own return to health in spite of dire verdicts, trusting that life can provide healing, and preferring optimism to pessimism—these are not denial. We speak too glibly of faith. Isn't doing nothing the truest faith? The truest faith says, "Your Honor, I rest my case."

If a doctor labels an illness terminal, the patient is expected to acquiesce to death. A whole new therapy practiced by some of our most compassionate doctors, nurses, volunteers, and psychologists has grown up around the idea that it is a kindness to help the patient overcome denial, to ease him gently into that good night. But hardly anything can obstruct recovery more than the patient's acceptance with good grace of the prognosis of death.

Certainly, in some cases, helping the patient die is a

great kindness—cases in which the patient deeply wants to end his tenure in life, yet is terrified of leaving. I, for one, believe not only that I have the right to die when I want to, but that I have a right to assistance in dying if I need it.

Yet, if my mind and body were operating pretty well, even though some tests showed I had only a year to live, I would like to stay away from the doctor who would give me the "truth," so that I could get my affairs in order. The doctor who would most likely help me get well would be "in denial" with me, encouraging me to be optimistic and advising me to get on with my life. Assuring a patient that he or she *will* die and mentally preparing the person for death helps to dig that person's grave.

Unfortunately, most of us think that the will to live means forcefully summoning aggressive emotions. A friend of mine whose husband died of cancer rejects any notion that the mind plays a role in whether the sick person lives or dies. "My husband fought death and dying with all his strength and will. He was always a fighter!" Like my friend, physicians point to all the patients whose fervent determination to live didn't keep them alive. The will to live, they say, doesn't kill a virus or reconstruct a bad heart.

Other physicians insist that the opposite is true, pointing to cases in which the patient's fervent determination to live was keeping them alive.

The fact is that people do die who want very much to live, who "rage against the dying of the light." And it is also a fact that people do somehow pull themselves back from the brink of death with what appears to be a sheer effort of will. These conflicting scenarios are not both right—they are both wrong, because they are both based on an incorrect premise. It isn't willpower that affects or fails to affect an illness. It is *faith*. Will and faith are contradictions in terms—they name two entirely different states of mind. The *will to live* should not be confused with *faith that one will live*.

"I will! I will!"—the very vehemence of the utterance indicates disbelief in the desired outcome. The will to live doesn't save and may actually destroy. Willing is stressful. Will competes with the disease. Will challenges the disease. Will fears the disease. Will depletes the energy of the body. Willing to get well is like trying to sleep. In one of his many brilliant insights, the philosopher Alan Watts points out that you cannot try to sleep. Trying is an act of wakefulness; sleeping and trying are mutually exclusive. The harder you try to do anything, let alone sleep, the more awake you have to be. Trying is a state of mental and physical effort: The muscles tense; the brain goes into its analytical coping mode; hormones fire the "be alert" response. All of these physiological accompaniments of trying are exactly wrong for falling asleep—they are also wrong for becoming healthy.

The idea that you can will-power your way to health is one more demonstration of the generalized violence of our society. We value aggressive competition and the will to win, and these values are reflected in our attitudes about health. We talk about illness the same way we talk about corporate takeovers and war: "A Fight for Life in Washington," "A Doctor Battles Cancer," "An Executive's Personal Fight for Survival," "Beating Cancer," "One Man's Victory over Cancer"—such are the titles of articles on health in magazines as diverse as *Runner's World*, *Industry Week*, *U.S. News & World Report*, and *People.*

The root of the word "agony" is the Greek word *agon*, meaning "contest" or "struggle." Struggling with disease is a state of agony. During the heat of battle, a soldier's entire being is involved in the fight. If your illness is your battle, it will not disappear from your life. If disease has become your focal point, it will *be* your focal point.

Will needs an object, a target; the effort of willing to get well not only holds the target of illness in front of your eyes, it also depletes the energy your body could use to heal itself. Soldiers may not be able to walk off the battlefield, but people can walk away from warring with their disease.

～

Sick people tend to take themselves very seriously. Humor, if it enters at all, is often the bitter and ironic humor of the gallows—not mirth. Mirth heals, as Norman Cousins so fortunately discovered. And his discovery initiated a new alternative health treatment—

Laughter Therapy. Now, even conventional hospitals have "comedy carts," which deliver funny videos and joke books to their patients.

The important question is, exactly how does laughter heal? If illness is an organic malfunction or an attack by harmful organisms, how can laughing possibly reverse the malfunction or oust the organisms? Cousins valued laughter as a kind of physical workout; it jiggles up the internal organs: good, hearty, prolonged laughing exercises the insides even better than a good jog or a good swim. And laughter releases endorphins—a potent well-being hormone. I believe that the most important benefit of laughter is that it takes your mind off your disease: While you are laughing, you are not thinking about being sick; momentarily, your illness has slipped from its primacy in your mind. Laughter works because fear and laughter, fighting and laughter, cannot simultaneously exist.

About six years ago, a friend of mine died of cancer of the breast. She wanted to get well. She wanted it so much that she spent most of her time working on getting well—she joined cancer support groups in which cancer in all of its behavioral and emotional ramifications was the topic of discussion; she delved into the study of macrobiotics and ate no food unless it conformed to a macrobiotic anti-cancer diet; she prayed to get over her cancer and meditated to get over her cancer; she read books about cancer. She talked and talked about cancer.

She did spiritual healing the aim of which was to cure cancer. She died of cancer.

Illness flourishes when we work on curing it, when we compose a little dictionary of "sick" terms to fill our mind and a story that has our lives as landscape and disease as the main character. When we make our illness the centerpiece of our lives, we are clutching it to ourselves. The way to get rid of it, to get rid of anything, is to open your hand and let it go.

Recently, another friend died of breast cancer—a young, intelligent, accomplished, deeply religious person who tried to heal her disease spiritually. However, her spiritual means was not a spiritual surrender but religious warfare. She tried to enlist the power of God, of Jesus, of angels to "fight" on her side. I single out Margo's case because it contains crucial lessons. As with the friend I mentioned earlier, Margo's body was a field of conflict where her will was pitted against disease. In her case, the conflict carried momentous religious significance—the forces of good battled the forces of evil. Yet religious as she was, she didn't "rest" in her faith. She believed that Christ could cure her and that he did come to her, but somehow, unexplainably, not with sufficient divine power to cure her once and for all. She needed him to cure her over and over again—every Sunday at services, every Wednesday at healing sessions. She was frequently "slain in spirit," and sometimes collapsed in a heap on the floor of the church. At these times, she felt she had been healed. But these healings apparently were insufficient, for she turned repeatedly to chemotherapy and surgery. During the whole of Margo's ordeal, the seat

of health remained outside of herself—a combination
of Christ and medicine—and she spent five years in a
frantic effort to make these outside powers heal her. Her
desperate search even included the search for a healing
geographical location: It could be her church building,
or it could be an airplane runway in Toronto where, it
was said, the Holy Spirit had descended. She did not
locate the spirit that heals *within herself*.

In addition to fighting her relentless war with
disease, she may have realized emotional benefits that
she was not consciously aware of. Because of her illness,
she was able to control the behavior and emotions of
those close to her in a way that as a healthy person she
could not, eliciting the constant concern and attention
that she deeply craved. Her courageous battle drew the
admiration and applause of colleagues and friends: As
long as the disease continued, she could be engaged in
a heroic fight; her flaws and shortcomings would be
overlooked and she would be bathed in sympathetic
understanding. In brief, her disease conferred upon her
a power and a glory that health could not deliver.

If a disease is permitted to offer such benefits,
how could it possibly go away? To be healthy, we have
to relinquish the perks of sickness. We have to give up
being admired, to forego a reputation for courage, to
want nothing from anyone that they would not give if
we were perfectly healthy—not loyalty or attention or
kindness or respect. We have to desire health as our only
gratuity, and to realize that the healing spirit abides
with us at all times and in every place. A Scandinavian
proverb says, "In each of us there is a king; speak to him

and he will come forth." Likewise there is a healer. There is nowhere to go to seek health; there is no one to seek it from—not God, Jesus, Krishna, Buddha, angels, or masters, for Divine Intelligence has placed the power of healing within *you*.

We are inclined to think that our conscious mind—our will—makes our choices. But studies of brain function have shown that something in the unconscious mind has already reached a decision before the conscious mind does its choosing. In *The Mind's Sky*, Timothy Ferris refers to the experiments that demonstrate this fact. One typical experiment measured the brain activity involved in flexing one's finger and found that there were two, not one, excitations, or "brain actions." One excitation occurred when the subject consciously wanted to flex the finger. But before that, before the conscious intention, a flurry of activity had already occurred: Something of which the person was not conscious had already been registered by the brain. That unconscious something may be the imagination—a level of function deeper and different from the willed act. This might explain in physiological terms why the will to live—an activity of the conscious mind—cannot override deeper, unconscious imaginings or desires. Ferris asserts that we mistakenly believe the mind is "running the show," when it is really playing "catch-up ball."[160]

Imagination and willpower function very differently: In willing to be well, you are admitting to yourself that you are not well; wellness may occur at some future time if you try hard enough, but right now you are sick.

Willing is a present mental action toward a hoped-for future condition. Imagination, on the other hand, sees the goal as present. A mental image occurs in this moment of time: You are well now.

"Through the creative imagination," says Napoleon Hill, author of *Think and Grow Rich*, "the finite mind of man has direct communication with Infinite Intelligence." And Montaigne says, "I am one of those who are most sensible of the power of imagination. . . . Why do the physicians possess, beforehand, their patients' credulity with so many false promises of cure, if not to the end that the effect of imagination may supply the imposture of their decoctions."

Imagination, then—the ability to see yourself and feel yourself as healthy—not willpower, is the mental state that can assist your healing. More than 30 years ago, the Italian psychiatrist Roberto Assagioli (see chapter 17, "Breakthrough Medicine"), who originated an approach to psychotherapy called Psychosynthesis, used his patients' imagination as the primary instrument in their psychological transformation. Through a variety of imaging exercises, he aimed to close the gap between his patients' actual self and their ideal, higher Self.[161]

Imagination can heal. It can also be powerfully destructive.

Unfortunately, magazines and newspapers describe in minute and vivid detail the particulars of disease, and TV and the movies show disease in "living color." A declaration of the mystic Joel Goldsmith bears repeating: "You can bring anything out on your body provided you are willing to live long enough with the idea of it in your mind."

The Simonton Clinic is famous for its creative visualization work with child cancer patients. The children are instructed to imagine the cancer cells in their bodies as ugly, repulsive monsters and to imagine the good cells (in whatever personification the child chooses) as driving the monsters off and replacing them with happy, friendly cells. As valuable as this process is, it contains a needless detraction. The problem with the Simonton creative visualization is that the "devils," as well as the "angels," are given great imagistic force, and the battle itself becomes interesting conceptual theater. It would be far better to imagine only the good cells.

The article on Hodgkin's disease I referred to earlier is typical of the way graphic description of a disease plants it in our imaginations: "In stage I the disease is still localized in a single lymph area; in stage II it has spread to adjacent areas but is confined either above or below the diaphragm; in stage III tumors have developed both above and below the diaphragm; in stage IV the disease has spread beyond the lymph system and has begun to attack other parts of the body."

If that is not enough for a person with Hodgkin's to wrap their imagination around, the article offers the story of Ruth: "Her Xrays had identified a large, dense tumor in the center of her chest . . . a second, smaller tumor, 'hard as a chestnut' popped out on her neck." Then Ruth describes herself: "I felt like a piece of meat on a slab."[162] Can anyone who feels like a piece of meat on a slab get well? I think not.

Name the illness and there is probably a support group to help people cope with it. There are arthritis groups, kidney transplant groups, heart attack groups. For cancer, there are not only generalized groups, but also specialty groups: cancer-of-the-breast groups, cancer-of-the-colon groups, cancer-of-the-uterus groups. These groups are formed with the good intention of assembling a community of fellow sufferers and can be very helpful. Group work encourages deeper explorations of the participants' psychologies and provides a setting where feelings can be disclosed without shame or guilt. But they can also be very harmful: The mere fact of attending a support group keeps the person yoked to his problem; ipso facto, attendance means thinking about the problem and group conversation focuses on the problem. Thus the group may help establish sickness as the hub of the participants' life. For example, one support group, called Living with Cancer, sends a monthly newsletter of the same name to its 1,500 members. If any of these 1,500 has succeeded in doing the best thing one can do—that is, living *without* cancer on their minds, the newsletter shows up at the door to remind them to get their thoughts back on the cancer track.[163]

"For those who learn to live with cancer," concludes the author of the article cited above, "the process is painful and sometimes exalting."[164] Those few words don't sound harmful; the statement even includes some positive words—"learn," "live," and "exalting." But what seems innocuous conceals invidious beliefs: First, the patient lives with cancer as a normal part of life, like breathing or walking. Obviously, the writer accepts the

prevailing and extremely harmful medical dogma that
once you have cancer you always have cancer—a dogma
that consigns the individual to an endless round of
follow-up X rays, CT scans, and blood tests. Second,
endurance rather than a return to health is the presumed
accomplishment. Third, pain is expected to continue.
I presume that emotional, not physical, pain is meant
when she says "the process is painful," but pain is the
reality she predicts, not well-being. Indeed, life must be
permeated with the pain of anxiety for the person who
thinks of cancer in those terms, for that person is cohab-
iting with a murderer. Finally, something about cancer—
perhaps one's continued victory over it—is "exalting." In
other words, in some ways cancer elevates existence. She
probably is not consciously aware of her implication that
cancer adds interest to life and makes heroes of those
who suffer.

The language of cancer is loaded with fear, unbearable stress, and victimization, and reveals how the
disease can conquer the imagination: "Whether one
survives 30 years as a cancer patient or only into next
week, the *struggle* is much the same—to *hold on*, somehow, to a sense of oneself as still being engaged by the
obligations and pleasures of ordinary day-to-day life,
even as one *strains* to meet the *demands* that the disease
imposes: how to *make it through the misery* of treatment,
how to *cope with a terrified family*, how to reassure friends
and *fend off* unwelcome advisers: above all, how to
survive the *personal uproar* that cancer sets off, how
to ride out the sense of *violation* and *separateness*, the

emotions of *horror, guilt, and fear.*"[165] (Italics mine.) The words I have italicized clearly exhibit the terrible state of this person's imagination. It is a perfect model of how not to think if you want to get well: The woman has split herself in two and settled into a continuous and permanent fighting mode (sure to exhaust the adrenal gland). Her life is a dichotomy; there's ordinary, everyday life and the cancer life that unremittingly underpins it. Her friends and family are terrified, and apparently she cannot allay their fear by assuring them that she fully expects to be well. She doesn't say whether she involves her family in her disease by describing her symptoms, her treatments, and her sessions with her doctor, but one can guess that friends and family would certainly be less terrified by an illness that is bland and boring. This patient makes her illness sound like an adventure. She would not have to "fend off" unwelcome advisors if she didn't broadcast her problem. Her sense of "violation," "separateness," "horror," "guilt," and "fear" is what cancer thrives on. She might practice using a gentler, more optimistic language with herself.

Schizophrenics' ability to put illness out of their minds—or I should say, their inability to keep illness on their minds—might explain why the incidence of cancer among them is only 20 to 25 percent of the cancer rate in the general population.[166] And in old-age homes, it is the patients who are mentally "out of it" who tend to live longer; their minds aren't occupied with their illnesses, thus they aren't stressed by them. Both these groups seem to demonstrate that the less your imagination is absorbed by disease, the less it will appear in the body.

In 1991, nine years after he introduced me to the metaphysical principles that inform this book, my ex-husband died of cancer of the larynx. He had believed deeply in those principles at a time when I still found them outrageous and absurd. But he believed more strongly in his sickness, so strongly that he tried every-thing to expel it—including excruciating rounds of chemotherapy and radiation. He accepted healing as theoretically possible, but he never really believed that he, the individual, would be healed by any means: neither conventional treatment nor alternative medicine nor self-healing. He practiced creative visualization and affirmation; he could visualize cancer cells being evacuat-ed from his body, and could sometimes imaginatively produce a picture of himself as healthy. But he admitted to me that he never, not for one moment, *believed* that he was cured. Belief—I use the word "belief" as a synonym for faith—is *the* most potent state of mind. The placebo effect is a direct function of belief.

In a contest between will and imagination, imagina-tion will always win. In a contest between imagination and belief, belief will always win. Ultimately, the distinc-tion is moot: When your belief is deep, you can hardly imagine something other than what you believe. If people believe that nothing will cure them, nothing will.

If people believe totally in the healing power of their higher self, they will need no other cure. Most of us live between these two extremes in a midzone of varying degrees of faith in various kinds and sources of treatment. The extent to which you can *forget* your illness, to that extent you are manifesting faith.

My revelation did not cure my cancer. What it did was make me happy. During the revelation I entered a state of bliss; afterward my soul was at peace. I learned that God exists and that I exist as part of the substance of God. I learned that peace and joy permeate the universe and were mine if I wanted them. I did want them. And I rested assured that faith in health was tantamount to possessing health. Just as virtue is its own reward, belief in health is rewarded with health. The powerfully healing state of consciousness I entered into was forgetfulness of the disease.

～⌒

Faith is not an intellectual activity. It is *felt* mentation. Total faith is not really faith in the sense we normally use the word at all, but a deep knowing—an acceptance of something as true with the wholeness of one's being. Most of the time our faith isn't that kind of "gnosis," but rather belief in the ordinary sense—a state that includes doubt, a doubt that exerts a pull against belief. But if your faith is a deep knowing, it is not in tension with anything. It is your *reality*. It is what IS. If sick people could believe they were healthy the way they believe the sun will rise, they would be healthy. This is faith healing in its truest sense, the kind that Jesus meant when he spoke of salvation through faith.

We can train ourselves to become better at faith healing. We can train ourselves not to pay attention to our health any more than we pay attention to the circulation of our blood or to the path of food through our digestive tract. If you were to listen obsessively to the beat of your heart, it would soon give you cause to listen. Let health be, and it will come of itself—in the same way that a forgotten name or the answer to a problem comes to mind after you have given up searching for it.

This self-forgetfulness is what I meant earlier in this chapter when I recommended denial. For if you fixate on your illness, you are truly "by illness possessed," and exorcism can take heinous forms.

The story of Nick Tanis as told in "A Charmed Circle of Survivors"[167] illustrates most of the destructive powers of mind I've mentioned in this chapter—misdirected support groups, negative use of the imagination, the ineffectuality of willpower, and the enshrining of the illness. The author observes, "Nick Tanis's cancer did not come at a propitious moment," and then quotes Nick directly: "There were about ten days in there—one of my aunts went into the hospital for a kidney operation, a very good friend was in a car accident and had his lung punctured, one of my students was having a pacemaker put in, a woman I'd known in high school went back into the asylum, and, oh, yes, another one of my students went berserk in class." Nick's life is filled with high drama, but I think most people's instincts would warn them to not become part of it.

Following this litany of tragedy, the article continues with an account of Nick's battle with death: "He has
passed through sieges of depression, hysteria and rage;
he has endured three weeks of radiation and almost
two years of chemotherapy; . . . he faces a lifetime of
reminders in the form of semiannual or annual appointments with his doctor." Yet Nick does not lack in
willpower: "Dammit," he says "I'm going to live! Whatever happened, I wasn't going to give in!"

Nick had been in psychotherapy for three years
before he got Hodgkin's, trying to reorder his emotional
life and improve his relationships. At the time he
checked into Memorial Sloan-Kettering Cancer Center he
says, "I didn't know I had two friends in the world. . . .
[Then] all these people started showing up at my door.
The room was filled with flowers." He asked himself,
"Who is this person all these people care about? . . .
There was only one conclusion I could come to: it
was me."

Add all this up and we can see that Nick was ripe
for cancer: He had had little sense of his own identity;
cancer gave him an identity. He had felt lonely; cancer
gave him friends. He had been alienated; cancer showed
him the sympathy of others. And now that he was faced
with a lifetime of semiannual appointments, his life
would be punctuated with little victories. His whole life
has taken on the theme of a basic survival story.

Long ago I asked myself, if ever anyone has been

healed by faith, why not I? If I, why not you? Anyone can find the healing I have found, and even more healing than I have found. Although eight years passed between the diagnosis and the surgery, I did finally have a cancerous lump surgically excised. Many have not needed to use an external agent of any kind.

You can learn to learn from yourself. You have experienced times when a cold went away quickly or when a cut healed without your worry or interference. What was your state of mind at these times? You can revisit it. Were you preoccupied with your cold or did you just forget it and go on about your business? Did you think about your cut or just stick a bandage on it and let it heal? If you can heal a cut, you can heal a cancer. The same processes are involved. The difference is that you are not afraid of the cut or the cold, and by your not being afraid they do not loom large in your life.

Faith healing is verified anecdotally. It is also discredited anecdotally. Stories like the following may seem to undercut the validity of faith, but they demonstrate only that faith cannot be forced: "Over one hundred people clustered around the altar praying, even begging God to heal a woman with liver cancer. The woman had six children and she was crying, even pleading with God to let her live so she could raise her children. She died a month later."[168]

A million people could have prayed for this woman, but if in her heart she *doubted* that she would recover, the prayers would have little effect—and the very passion of her pleas intimates that she did have grave doubts.

Dr. Barrie Cassileth, one of the outspoken critics of mind-body medicine, developed a questionnaire asking cancer patients about their states of mind. It asked whether they felt helpless or hopeless in their job, what their level of satisfaction was with life in general, and how they assessed their state of health. She found no correlation between attitude and the rate of survival or recurrence: More cheerful patients showed no greater capacity than depressed patients for fighting their cancers, and the pessimists were at no greater risk of death or recurrence than the optimists.

She concludes that the "inherent biology of the disease alone determines the prognosis, overriding the potentially mitigating influence of psychosocial factors."[169] Her conclusion probably afforded the medical community a huge sigh of vindication—conventional cancer treatment (and the hugely profitable industry founded on it) was on the right track after all.

But I must question Dr. Cassileth: Why does she respect the subjective opinions of patients when it supports her claim, but not when people testify to nonmedical healing? On what basis are the test questions valid? Ask a battered woman how she feels about her husband, and she will answer that she loves him. Ask an abused child if he or she is happy, and he or she will giggle and say yes. Ask an angry person if he is angry, and he will shout, "Of course I am not angry!" People shield from awareness their own inner states of distress.

Cassileth's questionnaire would have yielded more applicable answers had the questions revealed the impact of the disease on the patient's everyday life, the form their imaginings take, and the state of their faith. Had she asked the following questions, I submit that the answers to these questions would be profoundly revealing:

1. How often do you think about your health?
2. Do you believe that you have a disease that very well might take your life?
3. Does your disease interfere much with the way you conduct your life?
4. Has cancer affected—either in a good way or a bad way—your relationships with others?
5. Do you believe the cancer may well go away?
6. Exactly what will be different about your life if the cancer does go away?
7. Do you believe in God or some kind of benevolent cosmic force?

Earlier we examined the case of Margo—a woman who experienced repeated faith healings, yet died—and I suggested some of the thought processes that might have prevented her healing. I have not yet mentioned another very important and dangerous emotional payoff that illness may have for religious people: It may give a wonderful feeling of connectedness with God. The momentary sensation of being healed, the exhilaration of feeling that God or Jesus or the Virgin Mary or some other transcendent being has intimately entered your life, can become more important than being cured. One religious person writes that whenever "he felt familiar burning and tightening sensations in his upper back, he would say a prayer of thanks for his healing and the symptoms would recede."[170] He craved to repeat this ritual over and over to prove to himself over and over that he had found favor in the sight of God. If he were cured once and for all, how could he assure himself that his prayers were powerful? Spiritual healing can become addictive. The temptation is strong to keep testing God and to keep being assured that He cares.

Our culture plugs us into illness. Illness is comfortably familiar. Illness is less fearsome than a radical shift in our entire perception of reality. Karl Menninger once observed: "The sufferer is always somewhat deterred by a kind of subversive, internal opposition to the work of cure. He suffers on the one hand from the pains of his affliction and yearns to get well. But he suffers at the same time from traitorous impulses that fight against the accomplishment of any change in himself, even recovery! Like Hamlet, he wonders whether it may be better after all to suffer the familiar pains and aches associated with the old method than to face the complications of a new and strange . . . way of handling things."

For some, subconsciously, good health is as boring as a heaven in which all you do is sit on a cloud and play the harp. What can you occupy your mind with if not with worry? What can put zest into the plot of your life if not periodic climaxes of victory over illness?

Menninger questions whether humans can bear to be happy. Or is human narcissism so great that nothing but tragedy—heroic posturing against malevolent fates, proud martyrdom at the hands of a fickle god, or a speechless void—will satisfy us? In our society, the heroic tradition that keeps nationalistic wars alive may also keep illness alive.

The placebo effect, the effect with no external cause, the effect for which the synonym is "faith," doesn't jibe with our mythology of heroism. As Dr. Robert Heaney so acutely observes, there is "an American romantic tendency to esteem the battler who goes down fighting. . . . 'Quitting' and 'quitter' are terms of derogation. Somehow not trying harder is seen as cowardly."[171] It is more admirable to go down in the flames of illness than to slip inconspicuously out of its grip.

Let me sum up this chapter with the story of Jesus and the man at the baths. You remember that Jesus asks the crippled man why he has been ailing for so long when the healing baths are so close by. In reply, the man tries to convince Jesus that he is in no way responsible for his condition: He is not a quitter—he wants desperately to get well. Time after time he has struggled valiantly to reach the healing waters; but alas, feeble as he is, everyone keeps shoving him aside. Does Jesus empathize? Does he perform a miraculous healing? No. Jesus has no patience with the man's excuses and answers him curtly, saying in effect, "Quit your heroics. Give it up. Stop all your trying. Just pick up your cot and walk!"

19

triggering the placebo effect

I apprehend that if Greek physicians can cure anybody,
they do it through the mind.

—*Plato*

Item: Oxen suffering from a variety of ailments are
to be given a medicine composed of three grains of salt,
three laurel leaves, and three rue leaves for three days.
A cure is ensured provided that both the oxen and the
administering physician fast during this period.

Item: The healing of sprains and dislocated joints is
accomplished when the physician chants "Huat, hanat,
ista-pista sista domiabo damnaustra."[172]

Item: One of two treatments may be used for angina
pectoris: Either perform an operation that diverts blood
from another artery to the heart, or pretend to perform
this operation. Both procedures work equally well.

Item: Violent morning sickness in pregnant women can be stopped if a medicine is administered that actually causes vomiting—provided the women are told that it will prevent vomiting.

The first two items are taken from the tomes of ancient medical practices. But three and four are from recent studies on the placebo effect. Three is a study of seventeen patients whose angina pectoris seriously limited their activities. Eight of the seventeen underwent ligation of the internal mammary artery in order to improve blood supply by diverting blood to the heart. Nine of the seventeen underwent fake ligations. Five patients upon whom the real operation was performed were "much improved." The sham operation yielded an identical number who were much improved, and two of these five displayed "striking" improvement in exercise tolerance.[173] The researcher suggests that if an ethics committee were to approve a similar experiment with coronary bypass patients, they would find similar results.

In item four, the pregnant women who were experiencing nausea and vomiting were told that the prescribed tonic would eliminate the problem. The tonic was syrup of ipecac, a drug that induces vomiting. Every one of the women stopped vomiting.[174]

How can a sham operation cure an organic problem? How can a substance known to cause a condition cure it? How can "Ista-pista" mend a bone? There is only one way—through the mind. How can we get to that place of mental healing by intention, rather than by trickery?

When Socrates was asked how to get to Olympus,

he replied with his characteristic question-begging wisdom: Just make sure every step you take is in the right direction. The wrong direction for healing of any kind is pessimism and skepticism; the right direction is optimism and faith.

But how do you get to faith from here? Actually, you are already there. You already live in a state of faith—there is no other place for humans to live. You may not have thought of faith in this way, and so you may not be aware of where you have placed your faith. You can become aware by observing your actions: Your actions demonstrate your faith with complete accuracy; whatever you do reflects your beliefs. People don't act contrary to their faith, although they often act contrary to their profession of faith. In regard to health, most people have faith either that the doctor will cure them or faith that the disease will kill them, faith in their own weakness or faith in their own strength.

When I was first married, I tried for a year to get pregnant, and from the beginning worried terribly that I would not be able to conceive. From early childhood I had felt like an outsider, and childlessness would have cruelly proved that I was indeed unlike other women. I couldn't have articulated it, even to myself, but I thought I was not worthy of having children. I needed someone to affirm and help me, and I went to a gynecologist who told me that blowing air into the fallopian tubes allows impregnation to occur. I had faith in him and in the procedure: I was pregnant within two months. The procedure has since been discredited.

We already know that our society instills faith in

biomedicine. Alternative medicine attempts to shift that faith to its own procedures. Both are based on our faith in weakness and pain. How can we shift to faith in health and well-being? How can we get from bad faith to good faith?

Health practitioners are no exception to the egotism that determines so much of human behavior. Very few health practitioners recognize that their effectiveness depends upon the belief of their patients. Whether they are medical doctors, crystal healers, or acupuncturists, they believe that the healing power lies in themselves— or in the crystal or in putting the needle into the right spot or in the blood pressure medication. Ironically, their own faith in themselves and their techniques actually does increase their effectiveness: The faith of the physician stimulates the faith of the patient—a classical Freudian transference phenomenon. But the question that underlies this entire book remains the same: Why is it that acupuncture and surgery and a sugar pill can cure the same ailment? The answer points to the one constant factor among all the variables—the placebo effect.

In the late sixties, I became involved in the Women's Rights Movement—The Second Wave (Suffragists were first), as it was called. Women's Rights began with consciousness-raising groups. Neighborhood women gathered in each other's living rooms to talk about their frustrations and their unhappiness—most often from causes they weren't conscious of. It is amazing how most

women at that time unquestioningly accepted the role
of housewife and mother; it was the job of the woman—
confirmed by God, society, and nature—to keep the
house clean and the family well fed and healthy.

Most of the women had no money to call their own;
like their children they received allowances from their
husbands. They were unable to buy a home or a car, or
even to open a department-store charge account without
the signature of father or husband. The consciousness-
raising groups were not intended to be instructional:
They rarely offered specific advice; they presented ideas.
But when these ideas took hold of the mind, women
began to change their lives.

Likewise, a change of consciousness will precede
whatever changes occur in the way we handle sickness
and health. Consciousness-raising is what this book aims
to do—it gives you important ideas to reflect upon; it is
not a "how to" manual. Nevertheless, I will try to give
explicit advice on how to trigger placebo effects.

1. *Wake up to the amount of pessimism and cynicism
that characterize your thinking.* Most of us have learned
not to put our trust into very many things. We feel like
gullible fools when we trust. We have been duped so
often by the government, the media, the justice system,
the Church, and the people in our lives, that what we
fear most is more duping. And we have heard enough
stories and seen enough proof of the dreadful failures
of biomedicine to be left with little faith in doctors and
their treatments. We know in our bones that we have
been misled by the claims of modern medicine, but
having little knowledge and less faith in any "reasonable"

alternative, and having been taught from the time our milk teeth came in that without doctors we will die, we keep going back to them. The irrationality of our reasonableness doesn't occur to us: We tend to be like a man I know who was exasperated to the point of fury when a friend who practiced Christian Science died of cancer. Yet the same man accepted as an unavoidable tragedy the death of his own wife by cancer after she had exhausted all conventional cancer treatments.

If you don't trust doctors, though, you must trust *something*—or your chance of getting well is slim, indeed. Lack of trust coupled with low élan vital is perilous. Karl Menninger found in "a good many men and women suffering from cancer, an indifference to life, a detachment from life." No treatment can make you well if you are secretly tired of life. So, first, be mindful of your pessimism—bitterness, disappointment, displeasure may occupy your mind more than you know.

2. *Wake up to the nocebos that assail you on every side.* A nocebo can be anything, just as a placebo can be anything, depending entirely upon your reaction to it. But the most dangerous nocebos are those that are institutionalized. Outside of religious or quasi-religious organizations, our society has no institutionalized placebos—but it is loaded with institutionalized nocebos. I have already discussed them at various places in this book, but—whether you are well or sick—it is so important to be vigilant that I will list some nocebos again.

If you want to shift to a healing state of consciousness, avoid the following:

　– Support groups that encourage members to

continually rehash their problems and to share graphic descriptions of their disease and its effects upon their body. These groups also reinforce the person's self-identification as a diseased person.

– Creative visualization exercises that involve visualizing the enemy (in whatever form the enemy takes), even if victory over the enemy is also visualized.

– Advertisements and commercials that sell their product by scaring people into thinking that they already are or are very likely to be sick. Don't read them. Don't watch them.

–Religions that imply that sickness is a punishment for wrongdoing and/or a way to expiate sin.

– Religions that imply that sickness is a good thing—sent by God as a test of worthiness and strength of character.

– Movies, television programs, and books that describe illnesses, accidents, and medical procedures in precise detail and that make sickness, accidents, and disease glamorous and heroic.

– Doctors who practice "life-cycle medicine"—the theory taught to most medical students that health is defined by the age of the patient and that physical deterioration correlates with aging and should be expected. Life-cycle medicine regards ill health as normal and perceives the patient as analogous to a machine whose various parts wear out after a certain amount of use— what is healthy at 60 includes conditions that at 30 would have initiated extreme medical interventions. That a person can remain robust and healthy into very old age is a concept foreign to life-cycle medicine.

3. *Wake up to your nocebo thoughts. They're easy to recognize. They keep you up at night.* With the exception of excited anticipation of some wonderful event, what goes on in your mind when you are trying to sleep is a nocebo thought. Your mind may repetitively analyze a present circumstance, or continually recapitulate a past grievance, or keep imagining some future catastrophe. These sleep-preventing mental states stoke the adrenaline and cause additional harm that medicine has just begun to understand. You do not toss and turn thinking happy thoughts.

You can begin to rid your life of unhappy thoughts by becoming aware when you have them. Unhappy thoughts enter our minds as automatically as we turn the blinker on when we turn a corner. As with any habit, it takes practice and determination to change—a conscious, forcible yanking of the mind to a brighter place.

One of the most healthful states you can achieve is to become sick and tired of being sick and tired. Then you will discover that it doesn't take long-term psychotherapy to dislodge the world of unhappiness that inhabits your mind. You can dispose of it in the same way you dispose of trash, by taking it to the curb on collection day—you just do it.

I can virtually hear some readers' roar of objection: "You are recommending denial and repression. You are telling us to put a Band-Aid on a wound that will become gangrenous if it isn't cleaned out!" Well, yes and no. It is essential to be awake to what we are feeling and thinking. Psychiatrist Mark Epstein says, "When we refuse to acknowledge . . . unwanted feelings, we are as bound to them as when we give ourselves over to them."[175] On the other hand, we know the truth of "use it or lose it." That truth applies equally in reverse: If you want to lose it, do not use it. If you exercise an idea or an emotion, you will not lose its effects on your life. Continually rehashing childhood traumas, adolescent rejections, and adult failures keeps them alive and kicking.

When Karl Menninger expected the recovery rate to be low among people with weak élan vital, he was not referring to full-blown clinical depression; he was referring to normal people who drag through their days feeling overburdened, unimportant, and unaccomplished. Such people may not particularly wish to be well, because well or sick, they are the same old person in the same old life—the life that attracted sickness in the first place. Conventional psychotherapy might actually interfere with healing when it concentrates on familiar problems and their causes.

For just this reason, Lawrence LeShan has given up practicing conventional psychotherapy. I quote him at length: "A final reason I became increasingly uncomfortable with the psychoanalytic approach with patients with severe cancers is that at the end of a year and a half or so, I could see that the psychotherapy was having little if any effect on the development of the cancers. . . . They all died, and so far as I could tell, in about the same length of time as they would have died without the work we were doing." Traditionally, the fundamental questions

posed by psychotherapy have been, "What are the symptoms? What is hidden that is causing them? What can we
do about it?" No matter how well therapy uncovered and
worked through psychological problems that developed
early in life, LeShan found that "the cancers proceeded at
the same pace." So he began to ask new questions: "What
was *right* about this person? . . . What should her life be
like so that she is glad to get up in the morning and glad
to go to bed at night? . . . What are the unique ways of
being, relating, expressing, creating, valid for this person?
What has blocked her perception of them in the past?
What blocks her expression now?"

As patients became involved in answering these
questions, in discovering their individual "songs," the
rate of tumor growth was in fact slowed. After 12 years,
LeShan followed up on 22 patients who had been considered terminal and found that of those who became
engaged in the process of self-discovery—shifting their
focus from their illness to their unrealized potential
self—a remarkable 50 percent achieved long-term
remission.[176]

Unlike conventional psychotherapy, which travels
back into the past and moves forward toward the disease
as though it were the climax of their lives, LeShan's
psychotherapy begins with the present and moves *away*
from the disease into the future. If you use psychotherapy, seek out a variety like LeShan's.

4. *Be awake to your "faith" choices and expand them.*
For instance, you might acknowledge intellectually that
two doctors have very similar skills, but you would
choose the one who is cheerful instead of the one who is

solemn because cheerfulness is a trait that heightens your expectation of getting well. Another person's faith might be triggered by the solemn doctor.

5. *The dominant culture won't encourage you to have faith in your own good health.* Seek out small organizations that help foster your faith in health. These might be church groups, alternative medicine groups, or independent, upbeat self-help groups. Flee groups that teach the separation of spirit and body, as though there were two of you—your soul and the "dying animal" it is fastened to.

6. *Stay away from situations and persons that are toxic to you.* These are easy to recognize: You are not at ease when you are with them, and when you leave, you feel a lingering disquietude and displeasure with yourself. You can know what is bad for your spirit the same way you know what is bad for your body—it hurts.

7. *Seek out situations that make you feel good*: a gathering of friends, a walk in the woods, music, dancing—whatever is accompanied by good feelings while you are doing it and not followed by bad feelings when you stop.

8. *Explore alternative medicine, any form you feel intuitively drawn to.* I attach a caveat to this advice: Don't become an alternative medicine junkie, hurrying from one treatment mode to another. There are no panaceas. What you are looking for is yourself, the ultimate source of your own healing.

9. *Pray. Prayer is a type of autosuggestion.* God does not have to be persuaded. You cannot change God's mind by praying; prayer changes your mind. It clarifies and articulates what you want, and by doing so helps

you to deliver it to yourself. Some who claim not to believe in God (or in something analogous to God) admit they sometimes pray spontaneously or out of desperation. I would say that these people believe with their hearts though not with their intellects. God does not withhold anything from you and therefore cannot grant anything to you as a reward for praying.

Prayer is a powerful placebo, but most of us pray intermittently and lapse into habitual negative thoughts when the prayer is over. What are you thinking now? That is your prayer. What are you thinking now? The thought that can change you is the thought you are thinking now. When you can submit to the healing presence in the universe, which is available to you all the time, you will actually feel the flow of health through your body.

10. *Meditate.* Neurophysiologist J.P. Banquet says, "New sciences like psychoneuroimmunology, the study of the mind's ability to control the body's immune system, are showing that meditation can be used not only to prevent illness, but also to treat even terminal illnesses like cancer."[177] Actually, meditation is both a placebo trigger and a spiritual state. As a trigger it takes you away from the malady; it "detaches" you from your illness (and from all other concerns as well), and in that detachment or "forgetfulness," healing occurs. As a spiritual state, it can "provide access to an alternative reality." Meditation doesn't arouse faith in anything, but meditation is a state of union of the self with the Self.

11. *Acquire the habit of using affirmations.* Though affirmations are a sign of the desire to have faith, more

than arrival at the "place" of faith, they are a notable form of autosuggestion. In some spiritual disciplines— Christian Science, Unity, Science of Mind—affirmations are sometimes called treatments. The individual affirms that he or she already possesses what is desired. In a sense, affirmations are prayers of gratitude. They do not beseech. They ask for nothing. There is nothing to ask for because the affirmation acknowledges that whatever is desired is already at hand. Affirmations end with "and so it is."

Some people who practice affirmations mistakenly think of them as magical chants, as though the words *qua* words cause something to happen. Affirmations make nothing happen outside yourself. They make something happen inside yourself: They change your thoughts; your changed thoughts change your world. An affirmation is a tool to change your mind. When your mind is changed, the affirmation is no longer needed.

12. *Use creative visualization.* In the subconscious, thought often takes the form of images. As with dreams, the subconscious "believes" that the image is fact.

13. *Allow yourself to try direct suggestion for a physical or emotional problem you may have.* The practitioner of direct suggestion uses only words. If touch is used, it is used to soothe and comfort, as an expression of love, not as the source of the healing.

Direct suggestion is the method used by the Emmanuel Church. Early in their ministry in the late nineteenth century, the Emmanuels put their method to a severe test. At that time, tuberculosis was a common disease for which the only known treatments were a change of climate or the rest and special diet offered by expensive sanitaria—treatments obviously not available to the poor. The Emmanuel Church "attempted to ascertain whether the poorest consumptive might not be treated successfully in the slums and tenements of a great city."

The practitioner Edward Worcester would sit at the bedside of patients and quietly assure them that they were in a state of peace and well-being, guiding them into profound relaxation. Often they sank into a deep sleep, which Worcester believed was essential to healing. When they awoke it was as though they were following posthypnotic suggestion: They would be in less pain— even if their bones were broken. Or they would feel hungry—even if they had been rejecting all food.

"For eighteen years," writes Worcester, "our results were as good as those of the most favored sanitaria. Then the Commonwealth of Massachusetts, impressed by these facts, took over our work. Its physical equipment was, of course, far better than ours, but it could not command the faith, the courage and obedience and the cheerfulness of mind we had managed to instill into our patients, and it was not able to approach our results."[178] Direct suggestion directs the self to heal the self.

The great healers mentioned in this book—Mesmer, Quimby, Eddy, LeShan—all pointed to the source of power as the patient, and not themselves. LeShan, as we saw in chapter 14, concluded that the ability to heal was not an "arcane talent" but "a set of acquirable skills." If he could acquire these skills, he reasoned, so could the patient himself. LeShan asserts that anyone who can

enter into two or three seconds of absolute belief in
wellness has become his own faith healer.

And Jesus, of course the most renowned faith healer
of all time, said, "What I do, can ye also do." In several
places, the New Testament states that Jesus' power was
limited by the degree of faith of others: At Nazareth,
Jesus was "astonished at their lack of faith," and could do
no "work of power." Jesus' true power lay in his ability to
inspire faith.

In his important book *Persuasion and Healing*,[179]
Jerome Frank uses psychotherapy as the model situation
in which the placebo effect is brought into play. All
schools of psychotherapy, he writes, include four elements that are also present in faith healing, in shamanis-
tic rituals, and in religious revivalism. Psychotherapy
requires: "1) the patient's confidence in the therapist's
ability and desire to help, 2) a socially sanctioned place
where treatment is administered, 3) a 'myth' or basic
conceptual framework to explain the patient's symptoms,
and 4) an easy task for the patient to perform and initially succeed at in order to counteract the demoralization
that most patients have experienced in life. . . ." Frank
concludes, "One might view psychotherapy, in this
regard, as a highly organized way of bringing the placebo
effect to bear. . . ."

I extend Frank's conclusion to all situations in
which healing occurs. The primitive witch doctor may

catch the disease demon on a thread, seal it in a bottle, and sink the bottle in the sea. The New Age practitioner might write the problem on a piece of paper, burn the paper, and scatter the ashes to the wind. Biomedicine may dress the patient in a peculiar white gown and pass his body through a tunnel-like machine. All these rituals are part of a healing ceremony, and they evoke faith in an outcome; they play on the imagination and the emotions of the participants. Hypnosis, Hatha Yoga, Raja Yoga, crystals, creative visualization, affirmations, prayer—all provide lessons in faith: The subject submits to a higher power.

In this chapter, I have given a very generalized list of placebos and nocebos, but the number of nocebos and placebos is inexhaustible. For that reason, self-awareness is essential. Know thyself; know what arouses pessimism and a dark vision and what awakens hope and energy. Know what inspires confidence, optimism, and the emotions you associate with well-being. Know what arouses fear, pessimism, and negativity.

When we recognize that a placebo for one person will not necessarily be a placebo for another and recognize that we cannot control all the variables of a sick person's life, we return to the critical flaw in biomedicine. The scientific method *must* control the boundaries of the object under examination. It must regard the object under examination as a whole thing. But the combination of person/milieu/time that is involved in all healing is both dynamic and without boundaries.

Medicine asks *what* specifically causes this or that healing and it is always looking for a particular thing or procedure. The interrogative should not be *what*, it should be *how*. *How* does healing take place? This question leads us to look for the common element in *all* healing. This question acknowledges that there are myriad modes and contradictory means, *all of which* have resulted in healing. As the wise saying goes, "Each of us guards a gate of change that can only be unlocked from the inside."

If medicine can never predict what will cure a given person, how then can we ever rely on a given cure? We can't. But we can learn to know ourselves. *We* can trigger the placebo effect.

⁀

Galen was the scientific mind, par excellence, of his era, and for a long time he looked upon nonscientific cures as old wives' tales. Yet, ultimately, he acknowledged the superior power of faith. He directed physicians to "try magical remedies when all else failed and whenever a patient frankly confessed his belief in their virtue."[180]

Jesus' disciples talk almost exclusively of faith, and they do not always mean faith in Jesus, just as Jesus does not only mean faith in himself. When they speak of faith, they mean faith *qua* faith: the principle of faith, faith-fullness, faith as a child has faith, a heart willing to believe—an open heart. "Ye of little faith"—you who are the skeptics, the cynics, the jaded, the immovable, the closed-hearted—even Jesus would not be able to heal you.

One final word. For years I held the truth of my healing, like a poker player, close to my chest—because when I spoke of cancer, I was confronted by the terror of others, erroneous advice, and dire warnings. So, if you are stepping onto the path of self-healing, my final suggestion is to keep silent about your attempts or achievements. To paraphrase what Jesus said to the healed blind man, do not stop at the village, but go straight home. For unless others are embarked upon the same journey, they will be sorely threatened and will attempt to wrench you from your path with "facts" and fears. When the reality of self-healing has become so rooted in your consciousness that no other reality is thinkable, then you can speak.

20

the revelation

This book, at its heart, is not really about the placebo effect. It is about the power of God within. The placebo effect is simply the vehicle I have used to move beyond materialistic thinking about ourselves and our health. This chapter is our destination. To use the words of Michael Lerner, founder of the Commonweal Cancer Help Program in Bolinas, California, "It's not about curing, it's about healing." The word "to cure" comes from the Latin "to free from disease." The word "to heal" comes from the Latin "to make well." Curing an illness is not the same as being healthy. And the placebo effect is only one of the manifestations of the mind's power. The source of that power is God, and God's power shows up in our individual lives as health to the extent that we see ourselves as God sees us—as small gods through whom the Great God works.

Every year I commemorate the event of February 1, 1982 by holding a week-long personal sabbatical. From January 26, the day of the cancer diagnosis, to February 1, the day of the revelation, I retire from the outer world. I am obligated to meet with my college classes, but aside from that I leave my house only to take walks; I don't answer the phone or open my mail or watch television. I read, pray, meditate, write in my spiritual journal, *The Way*, and recapitulate the vision of Jesus and the revelation of God. I hold a kind of private Passover—reliving and celebrating the time when God entered the history of my world.

The revelation is the ground of my life. Not a day has passed since 1982 that it is not in my thoughts.

I had intended to retell the story of the vision and revelation. But I have decided instead to transcribe the events exactly as I recorded them in the pages of *The Way*, which I began on January 27, 1982, the day after the cancer diagnosis. Except for a few spelling and punctuation corrections, I have done no editing. Two entries were written in 1982, immediately after each experience, the others five years later, in 1987.

The second account, as you will see, is not identical to the first—not because I remembered the experience differently later on, but because at first my mind was overwhelmed. In the same way, one's first account of a violent storm might mention only the crashing thunder and bolts of lightning, while a later account might speak of shadows cast by the illuminated trees and the glassy sheen of wet rooftops.

The vision took place on the afternoon of the third day after the cancer diagnosis.

1/29/82

I read much of the day in Donald Curtis.[181] It's slow and illuminating reading. I feel the words as I read them, often closing my eyes and letting the full meaning sink in. I realize the meaning. When he says there is an "indwelling Presence of health whose function is constant," I feel it. When he says there is no place where God stops and I begin, that I am God, a piece of God, I believe it.

I went for a walk, up to the corner for milk, feeling like a piece of God.

I had a glass of milk and lecithin and vitamins when I came back. I don't know if I'm taking too much or too little vitamins. I do my best. Then I made a couple of phone calls—to Mary about the ballet program,[182] and tried to get in touch with Lee Barthelman about D.J.'s[183] stationery.

Then I read Curtis some more, and then I listened to a meditation tape called "An Experience in Meditation." It was a fairly good meditation, yet I wasn't so deeply into it as I was with Joan[184] yesterday. My hands didn't get warm and my mind drifted a bit. I told myself not to be disappointed, that there are all levels of response to truth and they all are valuable. Then the voice on the tape vaguely said (the tape was almost inaudible at this point) something about releasing to God, and suddenly I had an image of a presence,

not sharply formed, and something like Christ, rising out of
watery-like, shining circles. The circles were touching me.
They were like waves on a pond, starting from where the
stone is flung and rippling out farther and farther. The form
of Jesus stood in their center and the form had his hands
extended. The meaning was, "Give me your problems." My
voice said, and I meant it deeply, it was sincere, "I don't want
to burden you." The form became somewhat sharper and
clearer and the voice, very good-natured and with a touch of
humor, absolutely, irresistibly believable said, "It's no burden
to me, really." He meant not that he could carry the burden
but that when it reached him it became nonburden, nothing.
So I let it go. I felt that I was trembling, and I was crying. I
felt light. My body had no heaviness. I thought to myself, this
feels like levitation.

What I've written doesn't really describe the experience.
It was wonderful. A total sense of relief.

My burden was taken by God & it was nothing. Slowly
I returned to the meditation, and again my mind wandered
a bit. I was sorry my experience was over. I started to think
about hard-boiled eggs and became perturbed with myself.
Then I chuckled and thought, God has a sense of humor so I
shouldn't be angry with myself for thinking about hard-boiled
eggs in the middle of a meditation.

2/2/82
I returned to reading MacDougal. Shortly afterward, I
wasn't reading anything particularly gripping, I lifted my eyes
from the page & heard a voice in my head softly say, "There
is a God." There was a pause as this sunk in & gripped me.
Then the voice said louder, "There is a God." My mind began

to experience—what?—wonder & incredulity as the truth
of those words took me. And the voice said, a third time and
more powerfully, "There is a God!" At that point I was
seized—I don't know how else to put it—seized. It was a kind
of seizure. I was seized by God. A bright distant light sent its
radiance toward me. I should say, it was as though it was
distant yet it was fairly close—somewhere between 10 ft. and
an infinity away. My legs became hot & felt as though they
were being bound together. All the way up my legs, a circular
wrapping or rope of some kind, very warm, hot, but not
painful. The upper part of my body, arms & face became
somewhat rigid. Waves, like waves of electricity, kept moving
up my thighs & hips. I felt that my eyes were glazed. Very
slow tears, just a few, came from my eyes. My lips said, "Oh,
God! Oh, God, Oh, God," & I felt that some other language
was hovering around the inside of my mouth. All the while
this was going on—it must have lasted 3 to 5 minutes in clock
time—I was consciously aware, my mind was registering that
"This is the existing God, the One, the Real," (not in those
words). I don't think there were any words. It was simply
a fact—there was God & here was I. God touched me &
we both knew it. The words that were going on in my head
during all this were actually rather funny—they were, "I
can't believe this is actually happening! I can't believe this
is actually happening to me! This is too amazing!" Also I
thought, "I wonder if I'm going to survive this or if I'm going
to die right this minute." I didn't care if I died, it was just
an idle curiosity.

When it was over, many thoughts bumped around in
my head: continuing amazement. I was dumbfounded. Fear
that the feeling would fade and become unreal. I got up and

*took a step or two & said to myself, "You're still walking
& moving as usual. Isn't that amazing?" Nothing seems to
have changed. But what kept going on in my mind, with a
wonderment I couldn't shake was, "There is a God. I have
been touched by God & it is absolutely real. There is a God!"
At this very moment of writing I am still shaking my head at
the <u>reality</u> of it. I felt like calling everybody up: "Hello, Doris,
I just wanted to tell you, there is a God." "Hello, Carol, sorry
I can't talk long, I have a lot of calls to make. I just wanted to
tell you, there is a God. I mean a real one, a real God."*

    Jan 30, 10:30 a.m. 1987

    *On this day (the fifth day of the week) five years ago,
my little brother Jesus came to me. Curious that I should
think of him that way. Since the experience I have always
thought of him, & addressed him, as brother. Often, I feel a
special tenderness toward him, as little brother. Perhaps he
blends with Steve. Perhaps because I am older than he was
when he died, here on earth.*

    *On that day I was sitting on this very couch, though in
a different apartment, trying to meditate but feeling fear &
dread—the whole terrible material possibilities of the disease,
the burden of life, helplessness. And there came before my
inner eye a vision of Jesus. He was standing in water up to
his waist. Around him the water formed circles, larger and
larger, extending out out out into infinity. His hair hung to his
shoulders. It was brown. His body was neither muscular nor
emaciated. His face was nice. His arms were extended toward
me. He was gently smiling, calm, even matter-of-fact. He
said, very simply, nonchalantly, "Give <u>me</u> your problems." I
said, after a moment's hesitation, "I don't want to burden*

you." (It is significant to me that he used the word "prob-
lems," & I used the word "burden." His was a light word.
Mine, a heavy one). He smiled a bit more widely (not wide
enough to show teeth) and answered, "It's no burden." I still
felt that it would be, but I trusted him and accepted his offer.
All the time he hadn't moved, and his arms remained extend-
ed. I, too, didn't move but remained seated on the couch. I
reached my arms toward him through the invisible demarca-
tion between this world & the vision. Our fingers were a
hair's breadth from touching. I felt a huge weight roll off my
body, like rocks & stones rolling from inside my body, down to
my fingers. The weight never reached him. As it touched his
fingertips—or perhaps in the hair's breadth between our two
fingertips—they simply vanished away. And I realized that
Jesus does not carry anyone's burdens. He is in no way
weighted. He is light, peace, & joy. And I knew that to give
to him—our sins, our guilt, our sorrows, our terrors—is to
give away, to dispose of. Because they are not real. They are
our inventions, & this Jesus had come to teach, to show the
way, by taking upon himself that which is not the moment
is given away.

> *I returned from the vision feeling indescribably light. My*
body felt weightless. I had to look down at my buttocks to see
if it was really touching the couch. I felt nonphysical, and in
that state completely unable to have physical disease. I felt
cured.

> *Feb 1, 3:30 p.m. 1987*
> *On February 1st, 1982, near midnight, I had an experi-*
ence which changed the world. I emerged from it a different
person. It was as though new eyes were installed into my eye

sockets. And almost everything I had formerly believed was driven out of my head.

This was the seventh day since my new search into and reception of the ideas in Unity & similar books had begun. It was the seventh day since my operation.

I was sitting in my usual corner of the couch, reading nothing particularly different from that which I had been reading all week. Suddenly, & unprovoked, a thought—a small voice—came into my head. It said, "There _is_ a God." Somehow it astounded me. It was not a thought but a realization. It lifted me half out of my seat, & it came again, with more force: "There _is_ a God!" I was propelled out of my seat & a few steps forward with the force of the wonder of the realization. And it came again, full & clear: "There is a God!" My body moved more forward as though pushed from behind. The wonder of it, the profound _realization_ of it is indescribable. I was awed, overcome. I found myself back in my seat and the "seizure" began. I later described it as "being taken." I felt warm cloths wrapped around & around both my legs—wrapped together; circuits like tiny waves of electrical vibration coursed through my thighs & hips. The upper part of my body was rigid. My mouth was hanging open & my eyes were glazed. They felt bulging. I felt a great urge to mumble, the speaking in tongues which I have heard once or twice. But I did not. I don't know whether I said it or thought it, but the words, "Why me?" "Why me?" repeated themselves, for I knew this was possession by God & I couldn't understand why I should be so chosen. Then I had two visions, one in front of my forehead & one in back of my head. I saw, in front of me, eternity. It appeared in the form of vast churning & rolling clouds, extending into infinity. And I knew that the universe was ineffably beautiful, ineffably & absolutely Perfect. At the back of my head, coming from as close as 20 feet away & as far as the heavens, I saw a circle of yellow light, like an intensely bright halo. From this halo, a halo beam descended upon me & engulfed me. And I heard the words, "I Am Here. I Am God." And I knew that I was in the Presence of the Very God, Creator of the Universe, the Alpha & The Omega, God Who Is God.

I don't know how long this lasted. Perhaps five minutes, perhaps eight or ten.

When it was over I knew that I was standing on new ground & that I was a new person.

Eli Eli Glory be to God, The Beloved.

21

faith and the placebo effect

. . . the Lord our God, the Lord is one.

—*The Hebrew Shema*

What I have done, can ye do.

—*Jesus of Nazareth*

Jesus did not heal me, and his appearance did not induce me to take him as my savior. Quite the opposite: He proved to me that I was my own savior.

God did not heal me. He said nothing about cancer and nothing about health. He did not tell me to quit smoking or to practice meditation. He did not exhort, command, or instruct. He said nothing, in fact, about anything. He said only, "I Am Here. I Am God." Those six words and the knowledge imparted to me wordlessly in a roiling cloud-like, sea-like image that the creation is

an emanation of God, and therefore perfect, are the
source and ground of everything I believe.[185]

Over the years, answers have continued to flow
from the revelation. They come with the force of epipha-
nies in a process that usually takes the form of an
internal dialogue: Who healed me? *You healed yourself.*
How can I heal myself? I have no such power. *Yes. You
have the power.* How is it possible that I have such power?
I am not God. *You are not God, but God is you.*

Let me interpret first my vision of Jesus and then
the revelation of God.

Even as Jesus spoke the word "problems," it struck
me as inappropriate: Problems occur daily and we solve
them daily. I thought of cancer as a horror, not a mere
problem, and in a way I was politely correcting Jesus
when I replaced his unemotional word with a word of
great moment—"burden." My response showed my fear
of cancer, and it also showed that I accepted traditional
Christianity's definition of Jesus—the suffering god,
the scapegoat who groans under the cross of human
sinfulness. I saw later that my demurrer was both
magnanimous and disingenuous, and it evoked from
Jesus a deeper smile and a humorous expression in his
eyes. He used my more portentous word to reassure me,
"It is no burden."

Again I misinterpreted his meaning. I thought he
meant that though he did carry the sins of humanity, he
was equal to the burden. Nonetheless, I could not refuse
his offer, and I reluctantly stretched out my hands
toward him as though to transfer to him the weight of
my distress. Our fingertips were a hair's breadth from
touching.

The worries and sorrows of my entire life, not just the cancer, rolled like large stones from my body into my arms and down my arms into my fingers. To my great amazement, I saw that the stones did not roll onto Jesus. They evaporated; they vanished in the space between his fingertips and mine. They became empty air. What I learned in that moment overturned most of the beliefs I had adopted from Western religion, from psychology, and from literature—overturned, in fact, most of my prevailing beliefs from my society concerning self-identity, relationships, and health. I learned that no other entity—no thing or human or superhuman—carries the problems of anyone else: You cannot carry your child's problems; your friend cannot carry your problems; the scalpel or pill cannot take your problems from you. Only you can carry your own problems.

And I learned that nothing forces us to carry our own problems: We carry them by choice or by ignorance. The moment we have faith that something can free us of the problems—as I had faith that Jesus would assume them—at that moment they fall from us. But I saw that Jesus did not take my problems, and so I understood that we get rid of them by letting them go. We surrender them.

What I learned from the vision also adjusted my understanding of Hindu and Buddhist teachings about karma—the good or bad "spiritual energy" that each person accumulates by his or her actions and carries into the present and future. According to these religions, bad karma must be "burned off" by living it out. Irrespective of whether the person has become very different in heart and mind from the one who acquired the karmic debt, the debt must still be paid. Sickness, poverty, or misery of any kind are at the same time evidence of karmic debt and modes of dispelling it. What I learned is that a change in consciousness, whenever it occurs, brings a change in karma. To the degree that your mind and heart have advanced, to that degree you shed your culpability: A higher law is invoked by higher consciousness. Just as a person who receives a heart transplant from a felon does not have to go to prison, an old spiritual debt is not owed by the new you.

Proverbs such as "As ye sow, so shall ye reap" (Ecclesiastes), which abound in the Judeo-Christian tradition, like Hindu and Buddhist karma, imply that you must harvest in the fall what you have planted in the spring. But sowing and reaping is a misleading metaphor for the journey of the spirit. In the material world, a seed develops over time to duplicate the plant the seed came from—seed becomes plant becomes seed becomes plant. But in the metaphysical realm, in the realm of the spirit, sowing and reaping occur simultaneously; the person you are at this very moment creates the world you inhabit at this very moment. You couldn't, if you tried, produce the world you lived in last year or will live in next year.

When the prodigal son returns—repents—he does not carry the burden of his former sin of separation. If an undesirable condition from the past continues into your present life, it is not old karma catching up with you: It is the old heart and mind still within you. The present resembles the past because you resemble your past self.

In my vision, when Jesus said to me, "Give me your problems," he was inviting me to be the kind of person I had not been before. He was saying, give up your karma. Be new!

Bodily health is spun from spiritual health like a spider's web is spun from the spider. The web cannot be different than the spider is. If the composition of the spider changes, the material of the web changes. The web's material is not a product of the former spider or the future spider; when the spider changes, the material of the web changes. Likewise, your physical health is spun out of your spiritual health. When Jesus says, "Seek ye first the kingdom, and all else will be given unto you," he is not referring to a result in time. "First" is not temporal. Jesus doesn't mean first pray or meditate or love and then what you desire will be given to you as a recompense. "First" means "above all else," or "only." Seek ye only the kingdom and "all else" comes along with it, because the kingdom is all there is.

I believe that what I learned from the vision was the original lesson Jesus taught—the truth he preached when he walked the sands of Galilee: Your faith will set you free. He did not teach retributive suffering or his own surrogacy. He did not teach faith in him, but faith in God, and ultimately the faith that is underwritten by God—faith in yourself. He taught, as he taught me in those visionary moments, that to be free of burdens you don't transfer them, fight them, or overcome them. Faith that you can be free of them sets you free of them.

Jesus, I believe, tried to break the powerful spell

of fear, which had taken hold of—and still holds—the human mind. The story of Eden is, at bottom, a story of the birth of fear. Following our so-called transgression, everything in the world and in our lives became part and parcel of a terrible punishment: We fear our bodies, we fear the other person, we fear the weather, we fear our food, we fear our work, we fear ourselves. Most of all, we fear the God who did all of this to us. And those who cannot accept such a God fear the absence of God and the oblivion of death.

Fear has become integral to the structure of our thinking. Our individual fears seem to define who we are. Without our fears we would hardly know ourselves as persons and as humans. We even derogate people who have few fears; we find them unfeeling, "happy idiots." But our fears are our traps, the "nets" Jesus exhorted us to leave, the Satan he put behind himself.

⁀

The cornerstone of all the religions in the world is belief in an ultimate reality that transcends physical existence. All religions teach that union or bonding with this ultimate reality is the source of health of mind and body. My mystical experience—any mystical experience—by its very nature corroborates these beliefs. My mystical experience, on the other hand, wholly contradicts the dogmas of particular religions: their insistence that certain steps or rituals or ceremonies or beliefs must be observed before union can be achieved.

My revelation showed me that union with ultimate

reality not only is available to everyone, but is in fact inescapable. Union is perpetual. It is tied to no religion. It requires no specific act or gesture. It is there for you when you believe it is there. And when you believe it is there, when you carry within yourself the consciousness of your integration with the divine, then you are living in a state of grace.

Very few, I think, abide in a permanent state of grace. Consciousness of union falters; we slip in and out of our inner sense that we are integrated with the Most High. We turn away and return at varying intervals and for varying durations. But when union is realized, if only for a moment, in that moment health comes spontaneously and inevitably.

Ultimate reality is, of course, a way of referring to God. It is another name for God, or as Jews name God, *Ami Yot Ami*—I Am That I Am. God is the personal name for ultimate reality, and it is the name I will use from now on, for ultimate reality has shown Itself to me as a Being. This Being is conscious. This Being is creator of the heavens and the earth. This Being is in relationship with all of us. Ultimate reality *knows*, and It knew me. It "spoke" to me. It revealed to me that the material and immaterial substance of the universe is composed of Itself.

God did not come to me as an instructor, or a wise man, or a judge, or a loving father or mother. God gave me no answers. Yet the revelation answered the essential questions of existence: God is not unknowable. He reveals Himself: "I Am God."

Obviously God is not obligated to reveal His

existence. He can remain eternally hidden. Revealing Himself to us signifies our importance to Him.

We are in dialogical relationship with God. He hears us and we hear Him. We speak to each other.

He says "I Am Here." Where is "Here"? It is where "I Am" is. Therefore it must be everywhere. If God is everywhere, nothing can be separate from or different from God. "Here" is in every molecule, in every atom. "Here" is where you are.

The part of the revelation that took the unique form of a beautiful turbulence of pink and silver and grey chaos of cloud and water could, of course, have taken any form. The image was a concession to my imagination and to the power that that particular visual image had for me and perhaps for humanity in general. I felt indescribable ecstasy and bliss, for I knew that the image represented God's emanation, His substance. And I knew that everything that comes into being is made of Godsubstance, and I knew that the universe is perfect!

From those five aspects of the revelation I have extrapolated everything that at this time comprises my faith:

1. *There is no death, for the substance of God cannot die.* We are immortal. I do not know how our immortality manifests itself: perhaps as reincarnation on Earth; perhaps as reincarnation on some other plane; perhaps in a way I cannot imagine. No particulars were shown to me. I am inclined to believe that we can choose the mode of our continuation and that it will correspond to the state of consciousness we attain in our current existence.

2. *Although the Creation is perfect, human beings perceive it to be highly imperfect.* This disjunction results from an anthropomorphic view of the good. We judge the good in terms of our cultural mores and in terms of our individual pleasures. In God's view, all is good, for all is His.

3. *From the Creator's substance comes creators.* To be made in the image of God means that we are creators. Just as God creates the All, we create our individual worlds. The All contains an infinitude of possibilities. From infinitude we choose the particulars that comprise our lives: We choose our bodies, our relationships, our loves, our hates, our work, our talents—everything. Infinite possibility includes that which humans consider to be good. To bring these "goods" into the world, we need to select them, and we select according to our consciousness.

4. *Our journey is toward perfection and final resorption into the Godhead.* We move forward until the small god that is our present self is assimilated into God. There is no retrograde action: Life is a process of learning—living is equivalent to learning—and what is learned cannot be unlearned. During our existences, we achieve ever more union with God. Because I believe that everything in the Creation—a stone, a serial killer—is already in union with God, by "ever more union" I mean more awareness of union. Our awareness can proceed at a slow pace or it can leap to a higher level in the twinkling of an eye. Either way, wherever we are on the path, there is always a farther point. Those who have had a mystical experience know that the mystical moment cannot be

sustained; and therefore, Christ-consciousness, enlightenment, cosmic consciousness, nirvana, liberation, are
not absolute states. They are points on the path of a
continuum. Any point is relative to previous points and
future points—until the resorption.

The essential dilemma of all religious thought is,
of course, the problem of evil. Some religions
(Zoroastrianism, for example, or the Christian Bogomils
and Cathars—heretical sects of the twelfth century)
propose a second god, a god of evil, who is in a perpetual battle with the god of good. Other religions, such as
traditional Christianity, introduce not a full-fledged twin
god of evil, but a lesser though powerful figure—such as
Satan—who defies and hates the good god and whose
self-appointed mission is to separate the creation from
the Creator. The Christian model compounds the dilemma, for where could Satan have come from? And how
do you fight him without resorting to satanic methods?
Christian Science and other New Thought religions
resolve the question of evil by denying it exists. Evil is
an illusion, an error of perception, a mistaken view. Stop
believing it is there, and it will instantaneously disappear.
Mary Baker Eddy once said that if humanity stopped
believing that arsenic could poison, it would immediately
lose its potency.
My own conclusion resembles these New Thought
religious ideas, yet is quite different. I cannot deny the
evidence of my senses, and they tell me that by human

definition evil exists in the world. But I would die before I would deny the evidence of my revelation that the universe is perfect. It was obviously necessary for me to reconcile the conflict.

As I see it, what we humans call "evil" and "good" are part of the texture of the material and immaterial universe. I also see that they are patterns of tension without which the universe would be in stasis: Nothing would happen; nothing would ever change. The relationship between evil and good is dialectical; they clash and merge, and from that dynamic interaction comes a resolution that blends both. Evil is an illusion and good is an illusion: If we could transcend our humanity, we would see that the names "good" and "evil" are human constructs and are entirely relative—they reflect what we like and what we don't like.

But even though "evil" exists in the world, it needn't exist in your world. Whatever it is that you name as "evil" need not be there for *you*! You are the creator. From the infinite you select the constituents of the world that is your world. You design its patterns and forces.

By whatever name we call the Creator—Divine Intelligence, the Omega Point, Cosmic Energy, the Tao, Brahman—It created a creation that has the power to cocreate. It would be insanity to believe that you or I created the universe. It is enlightenment to realize that you and I create our own personal universe. God created the entirety—all good, all evil—unfathomable infinitude. I, a creature, do not inhabit the infinite universe; I inhabit a universe composed of my selection from the infinite universe.

The Judeo-Christian tradition allows that God has given us free will, usually meaning that we have the power to decide between two or more options or to take this or that course of action. But as entities composed of Godsubstance we possess a higher order of free will: Our choices are limited only by what we believe to be possible. What this means, literally, is that the events in our lives are of our own making—good or bad.

What has all this to do with the placebo effect? The placebo effect operates by faith. You believe that something will work, so it works. Selection is a function of belief. Having faith in something is a way of choosing it. Faith selects from universal possibility and causes it to appear in the world of the believer. In contrast, you obviously do not—cannot—select something if you do not believe that it exists.

In God's world there is a continuous *possibility* of sickness and a continuous *possibility* of health. It is you, as cocreator, who attracts one or the other. I cannot know, you cannot know, reality in its infinitude; we can only know those fragments of infinite possibility we are in tune with.

As to the goodness of God, what can be more good than a God who has created a universe out of Himself?

Throughout this book I used the placebo effect to prove that your cure is not to be found in an external agent, but within your own mind. To paraphrase Deepak

Chopra, thoughts are germinal events. As William James said more than a hundred years ago, "The greatest revolution of our generation is the discovery that human beings, by changing the inner attitudes of their minds, can change the outer aspects of their lives." That discovery is just beginning to take hold of the popular consciousness, and when it becomes the operative assumption, humanity will be immeasurably better off. We will learn to trigger the placebo effect at will, and the purpose of the practice of medicine will be to help us do that.

Now I must put the placebo effect into proper perspective: The placebo effect can result in a healing —it cannot produce health. A healing is temporary and attached to a specific problem. Health is a state of being. Healing is achieved when you have faith that something will cure what ails you. Health is attained by faith in God. A cure manifests a state of mind. Health manifests a state of spirit.

This disparity is illustrated whenever a sickness returns to a person who has been cured. The power of that person's faith in a cure brought about the cure. But if the soul hasn't been cured, if the person retains basically the same vision of life, the same fears, the same self-concept, illness will reappear. In chapter 19, I offered some ways and means of changing inner attitudes and thereby outer events. For example, I pointed out that imagination has more power to heal than will power. Now I must add this: If imagination is divorced from spirit, the healing it brings will be disease-specific and temporary. The flaw in creative visualization is that a person who suffers from disaffection with the world and disjunction from God can still have a vivid imagination. At the Simonton clinic, where creative visualization used together with psychological therapies resulted in astonishing remissions, the disease later reappeared just as it does when it is controlled by chemotherapy! I find the reappearance more amazing than the remission: The imagination produced a placebo effect, but the potency of the imagination, just like the potency of a chemical, declined over time. For a person to abide in a state of physical health, the spirit must be healed.

Like creative visualization, a placebo effect triggered by prayer is also self-limiting. Usually, we pray for a specific cure—"Please heal my child's pneumonia," "Please, dear God, heal my excruciating arthritis." Implied in this kind of prayer is our separateness from the god we pray to. If, in your faith, you convince yourself that your prayer will be answered, a cure will follow—but you will not achieve health, and the next illness will arise to be prayed for again.

God does not answer prayers. When you know that you and God are One, there is no one to pray to. True prayer demonstrates that you believe, as Helena Blavatsky put it, that "Existence is one thing, not any collection of things linked together." To paraphrase the great medieval Christian mystic Meister Eckhart: Between me and God there is no space in which to kneel. True prayer is an act of the spirit. Its purpose isn't to plead for a particular benefit—it is to heighten your awareness of your union with God.

Holistic medicine is far superior to conventional medicine in that it doesn't neglect the spirit when treating the body. Healing the spirit, however, is not one component in the healing of the body; healing the spirit is *tantamount* to healing the body. If the soul is healed, the body cannot be sick.

Imagination, prayer, holistic medicine—if any of these means or methods that brings a cure is not founded on a pervading sense of union with God, it will be like Hercules hacking off the head of the hydra: Where one head was removed, two more grew.

Lasting health comes from faith in our position in the universe—from conscious awareness that we are within what Teilhard de Chardin named "The Divine Milieu." Lasting health comes when we get our "bloated nothingness" (as Emerson called it) out of the way and allow the health that is in the universe to play through us.

It is possible to think of the placebo effect as a capability humans possess irrespective of God, a capability built into us by nature, like our opposable thumb or our ability to shed tears. It is the nature of the mind, we could explain, to initiate certain physiological reactions, and these reactions are associated with a cure. But it is hardly possible to conceive of constant health as a normal state of being—any more than to conceive of eternal life—apart from God. Health and immortality are possible because you and God are one—wave and ocean. Though you are not God, God is you. To know this is to live by grace. Health is a state of grace.

My own experience leads me to the unavoidable realization that enlightenment or cosmic consciousness is not an absolute. I was there. I was in the presence of the Godhead, yet I am here, still learning, still moving onward. I was catapulted in one moment into a state of enlightenment, which, had it been prolonged, I believe would have ended my life. But I did not remain in that state. I was returned to the world of relativity and to the unique point I then occupied on a path that is a continuum toward God. I believe I am now farther along on that path. I wish I were farther still. But I do not feel guilty about being where I am. I understand myself as I used to be and I accept myself as I am now. Knowing that my direction is toward perfection, I school myself to be patient with myself and to recognize my great beauty in the moment where I am.

Before closing, I need to say more about self-acceptance. Some of the people who have read this book in manuscript are troubled by the possibility that what I have said will cause people to feel guilty for being sick. "Isn't it enough to be suffering without being told that it is your fault?" they protest. Their concern misses the point. The feeling of guilt is a nocebo; it can induce or intensify illness. It is also a spiritual ailment; you cannot possibly have a sense of union with God and feel guilty at the same time. Accepting responsibility isn't the same as feeling guilty. In fact, feeling guilty is often a way of escaping responsibility: Guilt substitutes for change.

Accepting responsibility for the future does not require that you flagellate yourself for the past. The ability to for-give—an ability we all admit is a sign of a great spirit—surely applies to your self. "Fore" give, means to give before—to give before there is a result, before restitution is made. When you fore-give yourself, you give yourself esteem as you are now.

Guilt is a component of narcissism. It indicates that you cannot tolerate imperfection in yourself. Jesus' intention surely was not to cruelly instill guilt when he said, "Be ye perfect as your Father in heaven is perfect."

"What do you mean, be perfect?" someone could cry, "I inherited diabetes!"

Jesus meant that perfection is possible. Perfection is latent.

Accepting responsibility for our problems goes hand in glove with self-healing; if you are not responsible for your ill health, how can you begin to take responsibility for your well-being?

~

The mystical experience cannot be predicted and cannot be expected. It falls upon you. Unsought, it seizes you. So, when I speak of your union with God, I do not mean having a mystical experience, for that is beyond your ability or mine to initiate. By union I mean a steady, quiet, inner knowledge—a knowledge you carry in your bones—that yourself and the Source of Life are one. I could liken it to loving someone: The love is there, unshakable, in the deep recesses of your consciousness;

whatever else occupies your mind and feelings. I could liken it to drifting on a river in a small boat, knowing that the direction is the right one and that the weather will continue fine. Union with God is existential. It happens only and always in this moment.

This is living by grace. This is where health is: *not too hard for you, nor too remote. It is not in heaven, that you should say, 'Who will go up for us to heaven and bring it down to us, that we may do it.' Neither is it beyond the sea, that you should say: 'Who will cross the sea for us and bring it over to us, that we may do it?' No, it is very near to you, in your mouth and in your heart, and you can do it.*

I have set before you life or death,
Choose life, therefore.

Deut. 30.11-14

afterword

The purpose of this Afterword is to invite the reader to share with me accounts of their own mystical and revelatory experiences. Many of these accounts will be included in a forthcoming book entitled "Mystical Experiences of Ordinary People."

Since my own revelation, I have become convinced that mystical experiences are far more widespread than anyone suspects. They occur to ordinary people like myself, sometimes just once in a lifetime, and sometimes repeatedly. They tell us that we are not—as the saying goes (usually as an apology for wrongdoing)—"only human": We are more than human. A mystical experience proves to us that we are more than human because it lifts us out of the physical/material dimension of reality.

Let me describe what I mean by a mystical experience. I do not mean seeing ghosts, hearing strange rappings on the ceiling, mind reading, or participation in séances. Mystical experiences have been known by the terms "cosmic consciousness," "beatific vision," "illumination," "enlightenment," and "revelation." It may come in the form of words, a vision, a sensation, even a dream. Each person's is unique. Whatever it is called, and in whatever particular manifestation it appears, it is clearly marked by this quality: The person suddenly and surprisingly gains a knowledge that transcends their normal knowledge of the world. This knowledge is not acquired through the senses or the brain. There is no cause-and-effect relationship; you cannot insert a "because" or a "therefore" between whatever preceded the experience and the experience itself.

For example, if a person is standing on a mountain or in a forest or in his or her own back yard and is flooded with a sudden sensation of union with nature and a tender compassion for the surroundings, he or she would not say, "I had this experience *because* I was standing in my backyard," but could only say, "I was standing in my back yard *and* I had this experience."

A mystical experience need not involve sudden transport into the presence of God, Allah, Divine Intelligence or into the secret heart of the cosmos. The experience may involve nature, other people, animals, or any object. The poet William Blake says he saw the world in a grain of sand, which may be poet's shorthand for a mystical revelation. Here is another account of a mystical experience of nature taken from William James's *Varieties of Religious Experience*: "When I went in the morning into the fields to work, the glory of God appeared in all his visible creation. I well remember, we reaped oats, and how every straw and head of oats seemed, as it were, arrayed in a kind of rainbow glory, to glow, if I may express it, in the glory of God."

Here is another nature experience told to me by a friend. Some years ago, he was sitting on the ground in a park, idly watching a bug climb a blade of grass. Suddenly the bug became huge in his sight and he saw, as if under a microscope, every minute part of its anatomy and knew the innermost nature of the creature. This experience may seem trivial and even humorous, but my friend was never the same person again. He received knowledge, instantly and forever, that the physical world as we usually perceive it is not the real world. The physical world is just one face that reality presents to our senses.

Another friend told me of an experience in which she felt sudden union with all other people—everyone was she and she was everyone. She took pains to explain to me that she did not mean that she had an intellectual grasp of human interdependency—the kind that Charles Dickens includes in so many of his stories, in which, for example, a disease among the poor trickles up to infect the houses of the rich. My friend meant that she had an illumination that "I am He."

You can see why sharing experiences such as these is important. They make brothers and sisters of us all—we are all more than human. As *only* human we are Jews, Gentiles, Muslims, Americans, Africans, Italians, short, tall, rich, poor. But as *more* than human we are offspring of the Most High.

We rarely talk about these experiences. Our society is so thoroughly grounded in scientific materialism that we are predisposed to dismiss phenomena that have no scientific or rational explanation. We think of them as mental aberrations, as meaningless tricks of the mind, as daydreams or hallucinations or misfirings of the brain's synapses, or as just plain nonsense. We usually share them with few people, and we ourselves tend to diminish their importance—if not push them into forgetfulness.

The completion of the human genome project reinforces the material definition of the human being. For many, scientists, doctors, and laypeople alike, the genetic map offers the key to who we are—even including such qualities as temperament, intelligence, and talent. I feel it is imperative to counter this definition with one that emphasizes our spirituality. I believe that by sharing our mystical experiences with each other we will heighten their importance. When we recognize their importance we will change ourselves. When many of us change ourselves, we will change the world.

This poem by Robert Frost, the splendid agnostic, intimates the deepest reason why mystical experiences are important:

REVELATION

We make ourselves a place apart
Behind light words that tease and flout,
But oh, the agitated heart
Till someone really find us out.

`Tis pity if the case require
(Or so we say) that in the end
We speak the literal to inspire
The understanding of a friend.

But so with all, from babes that play
At hide-and-seek to God afar,
So all who hide too well away
Must speak and tell us where they are.

Our mystical experiences are God's way of not hiding too well away.

footnotes

Chapter 1

[1]The lab report of the diagnosis in 1982 described the tumor as tubular carcinoma. The diagnosis eight years later when the tumor was removed reads "Infiltrating ductal carcinoma. The infiltrating ductal carcinoma is well-differentiated, and in this biopsy resembles a tubular carcinoma." In keeping with my belief in the power of the imagination, I did not seek to know more about either kind of carcinoma.

[2]Throughout this book I use the male pronoun to refer to God. I do so reluctantly, for of course no biological designation could apply. The alternatives however—using he/she or s(he), or alternating between he and she, or avoiding the use of the pronoun altogether—are cumbersome or silly and call attention to themselves rather than to a non-male God. I say "He" only because that word slides by least noticeably. God is, as the Bible acknowledges, unnamable. Our language is sadly non-egalitarian.

Chapter 2

[3]Howard Brody, *Placebos and the Philosophy of Medicine* (Chicago: University of Chicago, 1980):8.

[4]Petr Skrabenek and James McCormick, *Follies and Fallacies in Medicine* (Buffalo: Prometheus Books, 1990):18.

[5]Lawrence E. Jerome, *Crystal Power: The Ultimate Placebo Effect* (Buffalo: Prometheus Books, 1989):79.

Chapter 3

[6]Lately I have seen the words "paradox" and "oxymoron"

used interchangeably. An oxymoron is a linguistic construct, a contradiction in terms, and may or may not reflect a paradox in the physical world. The sentence "I hate my dearest friend" is not a paradox but an oxymoron. It is not solved by changing your emotions or your relationship with the other person, but by changing your definitions: What do you mean by "hate"? What do you mean by "dearest friend"? A paradox, on the other hand, is an apparent conflict in reality. Saying that the placebo effect is a causeless effect is not an oxymoron that can be solved semantically. The paradox can be removed only by breaking into new territory concerning the causes and effects of physical disease and health.

[7]Petr Skrabenek and James McCormick, *Follies and Fallacies in Medicine* (Buffalo: Prometheus Books, 1990):18.

[8]T.D. Borkovec, "Placebo: Defining the Unknown," *Placebo: Theory, Research, and Mechanisms.* Ed. White, Leonard, et al. (New York: Guilford Press, 1985):59.

Chapter 4

[9]*Cleveland Plain Dealer* (17 April, 1994):4-H.

[10]George Dawson, *Healing: Pagan and Christian* (New York: AMS Press,1977):171.

[11]Richard Cavendish, "Bread," *Man, Myth, and Magic,* vol.3 (New York: Marshall Cavendish, 1970):331.

[12]Richard Cavendish, "Bat," *Man, Myth, and Magic,* vol.2 (New York: Marshall Cavendish, 1970):227.

[13]George Dawson, *Healing: Pagan and Christian* (New York: AMS Press, 1977):15.

[14]Malcolm Gladwell, "Annals of Medicine," *New Yorker* (July 8, 1996):37-40.

[15]Timothy Ferris, *The Mind's Sky* (Beverly Hills: Dove Audio, 1995). This holiday is also called the Harvest Moon Festival.

[16]Lawrence E. Jerome, *Crystal Power: The Ultimate Placebo Effect* (Buffalo: Prometheus Books, 1989):78.

[17]Ibid., 76.

[18]Ibid., 78.

[19]Howard Brody, *Placebos and the Philosophy of Medicine* (Chicago: University of Chicago Press, 1980):10.

[20]Ibid., 11.

[21]Petr Skrabenek and James McCormick, *Follies and Fallacies in Medicine* (Buffalo: Prometheus Books, 1990):17.

[22]Howard Brody, *Placebos and the Philosophy of Medicine* (Chicago: University of Chicago Press, 1980):12.

[23]Petr Skrabenek and James McCormick, *Follies and Fallacies in Medicine* (Buffalo: Prometheus Books, 1990):19.

[24]Howard Brody, *Placebos and the Philosophy of Medicine* (Chicago: University of Chicago Press, 1980):13.

[25]Ibid., 14.

[26]Robert A. Hahn, "A Sociocultural Model of Illness and Healing," *Placebo: Theory Research, and Mechanisms.* Ed. White, Leonard, et al. (New York: Guilford Press, 1985):181.

Chapter 5

[27]I use the word "primitive" to mean any society whose tradition of medicine is passed on by custom or word of mouth. By advanced civilizations I mean those with an extensive written language.

[28]One can't help noting that the elevation of the healer in ancient times and the sanctification of the healer in Christian times corresponds to the apotheosis of the doctor in our time.

[29]George Dawson, *Healing: Pagan and Christian* (New York: AMS Press,1977):95.

[30]ACTS:r:16.

[31]Petr Skrabenek and James McCormick, *Follies and Fallacies in Medicine* (Buffalo: Prometheus Books, 1990): 11. In 1920, Professor Eugene Steinbach introduced vasectomy as a rejuvenating procedure.

[32]Ibid.

Chapter 6

[33]Carol Ukens, "The Tragic Truth," *Drug Topics* (November 6, 1995):66.

[34]George Dawson, *Healing: Pagan and Christian* (New York: AMS Press,1977):212.

[35]Ibid., 213.

[36]Robert T. Divett, *Medicine and the Mormons* (Utah: Horizon, 1981):16

[37]If allopathic medicine has driven out all alternative routes for which fees are paid, you can imagine its

resistance to a route to health that is free. Homeopathy, for example, flourished in the US at the turn of the century, about 100 years after it was developed in Germany by Dr. Samuel Hahnemann. In the United States there once were 100 homeopathic hospitals, 22 medical schools, and 15,000 practitioners. But allopathic medicine won the day, and by 1950 the hospitals and colleges had closed. Now there are fewer than 300 homeopathic doctors in the entire country. The practice is slowly regaining ground. Homeopathy works not by diagnosing the disease per se but by regarding all the patient's symptoms and then administering a very small amount of some natural substance that causes these same symptoms. It is unlike vaccination in that it doesn't give a small amount of the disease itself, but a small amount of something that manifests the same symptoms. A typical response of an allopathic doctor is that of Dr. Seth Foldy, a family practitioner at Metro Health Medical Center. He says homeopathy *can't* work because it is at odds with the basic principles of chemistry. Dr. Garn answers that nevertheless it *does* work, though he can't explain how. Thousands of people can attest to its benefits for allergy, asthma, diarrhea, arthritis, and so on. I suggest that these infinitesimal quantities of poison are placebos. Laura Yee, "Homeopathic Remedies Can Work," *The Cleveland Plain Dealer* (April 17, 1994):4-H.

[38]Robert T. Divett, *Medicine and the Mormons* (Utah: Horizon, 1981):178.

[39]Flexner, *Medical Education in the United States and Canada: A Report to the Carnegie Foundation for the Advancement of Teaching;* Bulletin No. 4. (New York: Carnegie Foundation for the Advancement of Teaching, 1910).

[40]Robert Peel, *Spiritual Healing in a Scientific Age* (New York: Harper & Row, 1988):23.

[41]Ibid., 24.

[42]Ivan Illich, *Limits to Medicine* (Toronto: McClelland and Stewart Limited in Association with Maarin Boyars, 1976):26. These are called iatrogenic diseases: *"iatros"* is Greek for "physician," ergo, diseases caused by the physician.

[43]Robert Peel, *Spiritual Healing in a Scientific Age* (New York: Harper & Row, 1988):25.

Chapter 7

[44]The "materializing" of the human being has reached its apex with the completion of the human genome project. We have reduced our physical beings to genetics, a purely physical code that is too readily regarded as the source of body, mind, character, and temperament. Both soul and free will are eliminated from the genome definition of what makes us what we are. Please see my Afterword.

[45]Ivan Illich, *Ivan Illich in Conversation* (Anansi,1992):142.

[46]Edward Krupat, "A Delicate Imbalance," *Psychology Today* (November 1986):26.

[47]Ibid., 24.

[48]Oscar Janiger, *A Different Kind of Healing* (New York: Tarcher/Putnam, 1993):40.

[49]Ibid., 45.

[50]Robert T. Divett, *Medicine and the Mormons* (Utah: Horizon, 1981):180.

[51]The AMA rejects the anecdotal evidence of non-medical healing, but finds anecdotal evidence quite credible when it supports their own interests. For example, the AMA points with pride to a survey of patients that reported that 93 percent are "satisfied" with their treatment.

[52]In his article, "What Choice Did He Have?" (*America*, November 22, 1986, p. 317) Dr. Robert P. Heaney, a John A. Creighton University Professor at Creighton University, says: "It has been known for many years that careful examination of all tissues removed at routine post-mortem examinations often reveals unsuspected cancers. In fact, the prevalence of many types of cancer (for example, cancer of the thyroid, prostate, uterus) at post-mortem is actually greater than apparent prevalence in life. . . . Cancer under the microscope does not always act like cancer in the living body. This fact alone ought to give us pause about leaping too quickly to expensive, dangerous and disfiguring 'treatments' for something that may be a nonproblem." Of course, the medical industry's rebuttal to these facts is another example of the double-bind tautology of its thinking: The disease would have shown up had the person not died of something else.

Chapter 8

[53]My daily vitamins were one to two grams of C complex, a balanced B complex, 10,000 of A, or an equivalent amount of Beta Carotene, 800 units of E, balanced calcium/magnesium, zinc, and selenium. I have since reduced the amount of E to 400 i.u., eliminated zinc, and added 30 mg of Coenzyme Q10. Basically, I am taking a variety of antioxidants and immune system protectors.

[54]*Cleveland Plain Dealer* (17 April, 1994):14-A.

[55]This area is thought to control vital, especially sexual, energies, and its secretions were used in love potions and aphrodisiacs. The Devil is commonly depicted with a tail but it was popularly believed in the Middle Ages in Europe that he had no buttocks. The expansion of the gluteal muscles that forms the buttocks is found in no other creature but man. When a man stands up, these muscles encase, protect and conceal what is regarded as one of the most important single areas in the human body—the perineum. Near the human tail is situated one of the most powerful plexuses known to occultism." *Man, Myth, and Magic,* vol.2 (New York: Marshall Cavendish,1970):296.

[56]Robert T. Divett, *Medicine and the Mormons* (Utah: Horizon, 1981):22.

[57]Oscar Janiger, *A Different Kind of Healing* (New York: Tarcher/Putnam, 1993):100.

[58]Ibid.

[59]Ibid., 102.

[60]Richard M. Chinn, *The Energy Within* (New York: Paragon House, 1992):6-11. Dr. Chin explains the complicated principles underlying Q.M. Therapy: "Life is based on the movement of *qi,* so in order to sustain life, *qi* must keep on moving. But in order for movement to occur there must be something else to move to. . . . In Chinese tradition *qi* becomes more physical as earth, water, fire, wood, and metal. *Qi* derives from *li,* which is somewhat analogous to the Indian *Brahman,* the single supreme source of all energy. From *Brahman* arises *prana,* life energy. From *Brahman* also arises *purusha*

and *prakrita. Purusha* has no polarity; it is conscious potential. It instructs *prana* on what ideal or idea form to take. *Prakrita,* the second aspect of *Brahman,* relates to the *prana* of actual creation, the vital impulse to bring non-being to being. The three *gunas* in Hinduism are similar to yin and yang in Chinese; they are *Sattvas* (neutral field), *Rajas* (positive force), *Tamas,* the negative force. . . . According to the Indian view, without the *gunas,* no polarities or conflicting forces could exist, so no movement of *prana* could take place, and life as we know it would not exist. . . . From the *gunas* arise the next level of *prana* called *mahat,* or cosmic intellect. When an individual's prana reaches this stage, usually through meditation, there is an awareness of the wholeness of existence, but there exists simultaneously a subtle feeling of separation from *Brahman.* A lower level of *prana* intensification is called *ahamkara,* or the state of ego consciousness . . . the ego is experienced as separate from the world around it . . . conscious contact with the universal energy source is lost, and ego arises. This is the level of existence man is essentially 'trapped' in."

[61]Ibid., 84.

[62]The alternative therapies that depart most radically from conventional medicine are religious practices that Westerners use as medical practices, the ones that accentuate the connection between health and non-physical forces. Yoga, for example, although concerned with controlling the functions and processes of the body, is far more than a physiological regimen. The aim of the exercises and breathing techniques is to set up "subtle reverberations in and around the body, which find a response in the spiritual spheres and bring

enlightenment and power." This is the faith-healing edge of alternative medicine.

[63]In his book *The Black Butterfly,* Richard Moss identifies his moment of transformation of consciousness as the moment a black butterfly alighted on his nose.

Chapter 9

[64]Robert A. Hahn, "A Sociocultural Model of Illness and Healing," *Placebo: Theory Research, and Mechanisms.* Ed. White, Leonard, et al. (New York: Guilford Press, 1985):177.

[65]"The Art of Aging," *Psychology Today* (January 1984): 32-41.

[66]Robert A. Hahn, "A Sociocultural Model of Illness and Healing," *Placebo: Theory Research, and Mechanisms.* Ed. White, Leonard, et al. (New York: Guilford Press, 1985):183.

[67]A French Royal Commission investigated Mesmer's results and concluded that they were due more to his subjects' powers of imagination than to Mesmer's powers. This is yet another example of the way a scientific body, in its zeal to discredit one idea (hypnotism), blinds itself to an even more important idea—the astonishing power of the imagination.

[68]Timothy Ferris, *The Mind's Sky* (Beverly Hills: Dove Audio, 1995).

Chapter 10

[69]*Cleveland Plain Dealer* (17 April, 1994):14-A.

⁷⁰There is now a vociferous political push to initiate prescription drug coverage for the elderly and perhaps others. For a population already overdoctored and over-medicated, whom would such a plan really benefit other than powerful pharmaceutical companies? It pains me to take this position, for I have been a lifelong political liberal, but I must agree with Ivan Illich: "A professional and physician-based health-care system that has grown beyond critical bounds is sickening for three reasons: it must produce clinical damage that outweighs its potential benefits; it cannot but enhance even as it obscures the political conditions that render society unhealthy; and it tends to mystify and to expropriate the power of the individual to heal himself." See *The Limits of Medicine*:9.

⁷¹Muriel Dobbin, *U.S. News and World Report* (March 24, 1986):22. In Indiana, a grand jury indicted a faith-healing preacher when the patient died.

⁷²Robert A. Hahn, "A Sociocultural Model of Illness and Healing," *Placebo: Theory Research, and Mechanisms.* Ed. White, Leonard, et al. (New York: Guilford Press, 1985):178.

⁷³Ibid., 190.

⁷⁴Petr Skrabanek and James McCormick, *Follies and Fallacies in Medicine* (Buffalo: Prometheus Books, 1990):102.

⁷⁵Ibid., 123.

Chapter 11

⁷⁶Since the material was based on articles in the *Journal of the American Medical Association,* one wonders who the

audience was supposed to be at three o'clock in the afternoon. That is a rhetorical question. The audience is of course supposed to be you, and you are supposed to believe you are being let in to the inner sanctum of medical mystery.

[77]Stephen Gottschalk, *The Emergence of Christian Science in American Religious Life* (Los Angeles: University of California, 1973):146.

[78]Martha Fay, "A Charmed Circle of Survivors," *Life* (November 1980):122.

[79]Robert P. Heaney, "What Choice Did He Have?" *America* (November 22, 1986):317.

[80]A.S. St. Leger. "The Anomaly That Wouldn't Go Away," *Lancet* 2 (November 25, 1978):32.

Chapter 12

[81]Robert P. Heaney, "What Choice Did He Have?" *America* (November 22, 1986):318.

[82]Ibid., 319.

[83]Exodus 15:26.

[84]Petr Skrabanek and James McCormick, *Follies and Fallacies in Medicine* (Buffalo: Prometheus Books, 1990):69.

[85]I can certainly testify to the deep compassion and concern of my physician daughter-in-law and sister-in-law.

Chapter 13

[86]Fred M.Frohock, *Healing Powers: Alternative Medicine, Spiritual Communities, and the State* (Chicago: University

of Chicago, 1992):130. The body's ability to grow alternative blood vessels is not as uncommon as it seems. Among the body's "wisdoms" is the creation of redundant systems. But it is enormously uncommon to find blood vessels appearing overnight.

[87]George Dawson, *Healing: Pagan and Christian* (New York: AMS Press, 1977):106.

[88]It is my dear hope that this book will encourage people to form groups where self-healers can gather, share their experiences, and rejoice.

[89]Wisdom of Jesus Son of Sirach:38:1.

[90]I use Unity to exemplify other New Thought religions—Divine Science, Science of Mind, Religious Science. It was the writings of the gurus of the "science religions"—Myrtle and John Fillmore, Emma Curtis Hopkins, Ernest Holmes, Thomas Troward, Don Curtis, Eric Butterworth, Kathryn McDougal—that prepared me for the revelation that changed my life completely and forever.

[91]This is actually precisely what Quimby taught. Eddy differentiates her ideas from his by emphasizing Jesus and Christianity.

[92]See M.B. Eddy's 32-point "platform," which outlines the principles of "divine metaphysics" in *Science and Health with a Key to the Scriptures* (The First Church of Christ, Scientist, 1934):330-340.

[93]*Man, Myth, and Magic,* Vol. 3 (New York: Marshall Cavendish, 1970):286.

[94]Hinduism teaches the five principles of nature, the first of which, the soniferous ether, or *akasha,* is all pervading and is responsible for light and sound. Theosophists speak of the Akashic Record—an energy envelope, that holds the impressions of all events, actions, thoughts. For a contemporary version of this idea see Rupert Sheldrake's *The Presence of the Past.*

[95]James Dillett Freeman, *The Story of Unity* (Unity Village: Unity Books, 1978):40.

[96]Ibid., 49 and passim.

[97]Theosophy does not hold itself to be a religion but rather a belief system and a practice, available to anyone in any religion. I quote from a letter to me from John Algeo, president of the Theosophical Society in America: "We are concerned with ultimate values, and that is typically a religious concern, but I don't know any Theosophists who would answer 'Theosophy' if asked what their religion is. We have members who are Christians, Jews, Muslims, Hindus, Buddhists, Zoroastrians, and what not. . . .We are a way of looking at the world, so might be called a philosophy, I suppose, but generally we think we do not quite fit into any of the conventional categories of that type. In a sense we are a religious philosophy. Unity, called the 'School' of Christianity, and, abjuring dogma of all kinds, is equally welcoming of all who practice other religions."

[98]Melville, Herman, *The Confidence Man: His Masquerade* (New York: 1961):98.

[99]I owe the metaphysical interpretation of *The Wizard of Oz* to Dr. John Algeo, professor emeritus, University

of Georgia, and president of the American Linquist Association. He is also the president of the American Theosophical Society. He points out that the theme of *The Wizard of Oz* is identical to that of most fairy tales and most myths: a journey from "here" to "there" in search of something wonderful and perfect. The seeking self goes out to find that which it lacks and is returned to what it has always had. The circle ends, after much hardship and travail, where it began, at the point of the holy self, the Atman.

[100]Red M. Frohock, *Healing Powers: Alternative Medicine, Spiritual Communities, and the State* (Chicago: University of Chicago, 1992):2.

[101]*Man, Myth, and Magic,* vol.3 (New York: Marshall Cavendish, 1970):388.

[102]Fred M. Frohock, *Healing Powers: Alternative Medicine, Spiritual Communities, and the State* (Chicago: University of Chicago, 1992):229.

[103]Ibid., 228.

[104]Ibid., 213.

[105]Howard Brody, *Placebos and the Philosophy of Medicine* (Chicago: University of Chicago Press, 1980):23. Quoting T. Findley, "The Placebo and the Physician," *Medical Clinics of North America* 37:182-23.

Chapter 14

[106]It is thought that some ulcers may be caused by viruses or bacteria.

[107]Robert A. Hahn, "A Sociocultural Model of Illness and

Healing," *Placebo: Theory Research, and Mechanisms.* Ed. White, Leonard, et al. (New York: Guilford Press, 1985):175.

[108]Leon Jaroff, "Can Attitudes Affect Cancer?" *Time* (June 24, 1985):69.

[109]Ibid.

[110]Larry Dossey, *Recovering the Soul* (Bantam Doubleday Dell Audio, 1989).

[111]I have a great deal of trouble with the idea that prayer is effective even when the patient is not aware he is being prayed for. What is the source of the potency? There is no intrinsic magic in the words of prayer. There is no inherent power in the person uttering the prayer. I do not believe that one person can manipulate the state of being of another without the other's consent. And who is being prayed to—God? Or an amorphous "force in the universe"? And is that God or that force so stubborn that it withholds health unless it is beseeched? Prayer does, in fact, work. But it works only when the patient participates in it in some way; it works not because something called prayer is being done, but because knowing one is being prayed for can evoke a host of healing feelings and thoughts and helps to instill faith in the patient. It is the faith that cures. The only basis upon which I can accept the idea that unknown prayer works is that the patient and the one praying are linked by some sort of ESP or by some other metaphysical force. This possibility is in fact the theme of Dr. Dossey's latest book, *Reinventing Medicine.* He presents a theory of "non-local mind," which I interpret as a type of PSI phenomenon that puts

one mind in touch with the thoughts of another.

[112]Lawrence E. Jerome, *Crystal Power: The Ultimate Placebo Effect* (Buffalo: Prometheus Books, 1989):86.

[113]Ibid., 101.

Chapter 15

[114]Please see the Afterword, in which I invite the reader to send me accounts of his or her own mystical experiences.

[115]*A Century of Christian Science Healing* (Boston: Christian Science Publishing Society, 1966):93.

[116]Robert T. Divett, *Medicine and the Mormons* (Utah: Horizon, 1981):41.

[117]Ibid., 43.

[118]Elwood Worchester and Samuel McComb, *Body, Mind, and Spirit* (Boston: Marshall Jones, 1931):208.

[119]Oscar Janiger, *A Different Kind of Healing* (New York: Tarcher/Putnam, 1993):36.

[120]Brugh Joy, *Joy's Way* (Los Angeles: J.P. Tarcher:1979) 208-9.

[121]Elwood Worchester and Samuel McComb, *Body, Mind, and Spirit* (Boston: Marshall Jones, 1931):29.

[122]Harmon H. Bro, *Edgar Cayce on Dreams* (New York: Warner Books,1968): passim.

[123]Robert P. Heaney, "What Choice Did He Have?" *America* (November 22, 1986):316.

Chapter 16

[124]Harold H. Bloomfield and Kory, *Transcendental Meditation* (Boston: GK Hall, 1976):337. Important experiments were conducted as early as the 1930s in India at the Twenty-Sixth International Congress of the Physiological Sciences, which are only now gaining credibility, and even now among a small fraction of physicians. Among the small number who are most interested in the role of the mind in illness, I could name Dr. Alvin Tarlogg, Director of the Texas Institute for Society and Population Health; Dr. James Gordon, Director of the Center for Mind-Body Medicine in Washington, D.C.; Dr. Esther Sternberg, author of *The Balance Within;* Dr. Barry Bitman, neurologist, The Mind Body Wellness Center in Meadville, PA; Dr. David Siegel, psychiatrist, Stanford University.

[125]Oscar Janiger, *A Different Kind of Healing* (New York: Tarcher/Putnam, 1993):59.

[126]I repeat my objection to the partitioning of the human being. While the approach of doctors like Kinderlehrer is certainly a giant step in the right direction, the language of division, naming the aspects, makes us think that aspects are parts that actually exist and that are qualitatively different from one another. Is there a director of this cast of characters? I'm inclined to believe that the structure of a human entity is analogous to multiple personality syndrome—now one and now another character steps forth—sometimes the character "organic," sometimes the character "biochemical," etc., depending upon what the observer is looking for.

[127]Howard Brody, *Placebos and the Philosophy of Medicine* (Chicago: University of Chicago Press, 1980):11.

[128]George Dawson, *Healing: Pagan and Christian* (New York: AMS Press,1977):286.

[129]Robert A. Hahn, "A Sociocultural Model of Illness and Healing," *Placebo: Theory Research, and Mechanisms.* Ed. White, Leonard, et al. (New York: Guilford Press, 1985):178.

[130]Howard Brody, *Placebos and the Philosophy of Medicine* (Chicago: University of Chicago Press, 1980):1.

[131]Jon D. Levine and Newton C. Gordon, "Growing Pains in Psychobiological Research," *Placebo: Theory Research, and Mechanisms.* Ed. White, Leonard, et al. (New York: Guilford Press, 1985):398.

[132]Howard Brody, *Placebos and the Philosophy of Medicine* (Chicago: University of Chicago Press, 1980):18.

[133]Brugh Joy, *Joy's Way* (Los Angeles: J.P. Tarcher:1979):52.

[134]Rupert Sheldrake, *The Presence of the Past* (New York: Vintage,1989): passim.

[135]My revelation showed me that all that is was originally and is ultimately an emanation of God. This leads me to one ontological conclusion—monism. Monism is also the most plausible explanation of the relationship between the material and immaterial dimensions of reality. If they are not one, we cannot escape from the dilemma symbolized by the expulsion from Eden; we will either denigrate and abuse the body or denigrate and abuse the soul.

[136]Elwood Worchester and Samuel McComb, *Body, Mind, and Spirit* (Boston: Marshall Jones, 1931):15.

[137]George Dawson, *Healing: Pagan and Christian* (New York: AMS Press,1977):287. Quoting *British Medical Journal*, Oct 1, 1910.

[138]Ibid., 287.

[139]Oscar Janiger, *A Different Kind of Healing* (New York: Tarcher/Putnam, 1993):180.

[140]Harold Bloomfield and Robert B. Kory, *TM:Transcendental Meditation* (Boston: GK Hall, 1976):331.

[141]Nancy Shulins, "Trauma Leaves Biological Clues," *Plain Dealer* (November 17, 1996):1-j.

Chapter 17

[142]Oscar Janiger, *A Different Kind of Healing* (New York: Tarcher/Putnam, 1993):32.

[143]Ibid., 53.

[144]Petr Skrabenek and James McCormick, *Follies and Fallacies in Medicine* (Buffalo: Prometheus Books, 1990):24.

[145]*Fashion: A Publication of Toronto Life* (May 2000):87.

[146]Mark Gottlieb, "Imagine," *CWRU Magazine* (February 1996):30-34.

[147]Fred M.Frohock, *Healing Powers: Alternative Medicine, Spiritual Communities, and the State* (Chicago: University of Chicago, 1992):198.

[148]T.D. Borkovec, "Placebo: Defining the Unknown,"

Placebo: Theory Research, and Mechanisms. Ed. White, Leonard, et al. (New York: Guilford Press, 1985):59.

[149]Oscar Janiger, *A Different Kind of Healing* (New York: Tarcher/Putnam, 1993):168.

[150]Ibid., 173.

[151]Ibid., 178.

[152]Ibid., 180.

[153]George Dawson, *Healing: Pagan and Christian* (New York: AMS Press,1977):288.

[154]And vice versa; the mind can be approached through the body, e.g., the work of Moshe Feldenkrais, Wilhelm Reich, and others, as mentioned in chapter 16, "The Physiology of Faith."

[155]Viktor Frankl developed this psychological theory during his internment in a Nazi death camp. He attributed his survival to his spiritual attachment to his beloved wife, whose soul seemed present to him during the misery of his incarceration.

[156]It has been found that though creative visualization seems to work wonders at the beginning of cancer treatment, its benefits do not last. I will deal with this issue in the last chapter of the book.

[157]Brugh Joy, *Joy's Way* (Los Angeles: J.P. Tarcher, 1979): 129.

[158]George Dawson, *Healing: Pagan and Christian* (New York: AMS Press, 1977):227.

[159]Petr Skrabanek and James McCormick, *Follies and Fallacies in Medicine* (Buffalo: Prometheus Books, 1990):21.

Chapter 18

[160]We have all experienced this sort of phenomenon in connection with our emotions. If we are passionately in love and are asked why we love this person, the logical mind immediately goes into action and begins to make up reasons, but the heart knows the reasons do not account for the love.

[161]Roberto Assagioli, *Psychosynthesis: A Manual of Principles and Techniques.* (New York: Hobbs, Dorman, 1965) (passim).

[162]Martha Fay, "A Charmed Circle of Survivors," *Life* (November 1980):122.

[163]Ibid., 126.

[164]Ibid., 121.

[165]Ibid., 121.

[166]Richard Moss, *The Black Butterfly: An Invitation to Radical Aliveness* (Berkeley: Celestial Arts, 1986):33.

[167]Martha Fay, "A Charmed Circle of Survivors," *Life* (November 1980):128-30.

[168]Fred M. Frohock, *Healing Powers: Alternative Medicine, Spiritual Communities, and the State* (Chicago: University of Chicago, 1992):55.

[169]Leon Jaroff, "Can Attitude Affect Cancer?" *Time* (June 24, 1985):69.

[170]Roberta Hubbard, "Gift of the Spirit," *CWRU Magazine* (May 1995):34.

[171]Robert P. Heaney, "What Choice Did He Have?" *America* (November 22, 1986):320.

Chapter 19

[172]George Dawson, *Healing: Pagan and Christian* (New York: AMS Press, 1977):85.

[173]Adolf Grunbaum, "Explication and Implications of the Placebo Concept," *Placebo: Theory Research, and Mechanisms.* Ed. White, Leonard, et al. (New York: Guilford Press, 1985):29-30. On the subject of successful sham coronary surgery, see also Petr Skrabanek and James McCormick, *Follies and Fallacies in Medicine* (Buffalo: Prometheus Books, 1990):19.

[174]This was the experiment that convinced Dr. Benson to look more deeply into the placebo effect and all of its implications related to the role of the mind in the health of the body.

[175]Mark Epstein, *Thoughts Without a Thinker* (New York: Basic Books, 1995):24.

[176]Fred M. Frohock, *Healing Powers: Alternative Medicine, Spiritual Communities, and the State* (Chicago: University of Chicago, 1992):199-202.

[177]Richard M. Chinn, *The Energy Within* (New York: Paragon House, 1992):107.

[178]Elwood Worchester and Samuel McComb, *Body, Mind, and Spirit* (Boston: Marshall Jones, 1931):15.

[179]Jerome Frank, *Persuasion and Healing* (New York: Schocken Books, 1974):325-30.

[180]George Dawson, *Healing: Pagan and Christian* (New York: AMS Press,1977):191.

Chapter 20

[181]Donald Curtis, *Your Thoughts Can Change Your Life* (No. Hollywood, Wilshire Book Company, 1979).

[182]Mary is my friend Mary Chadbourne. She and I were putting together a program called "Word Moves," (sponsored by the Poets League of Greater Cleveland), in which dancers accompanied the spoken word of poetry.

[183]D.J. is Donald Joseph Kuby, my former husband.

[184]The tape was by Kathryn McDougal. Joan is Joan Gattuso, then minister of Unity of Mt. Chalet, now minister of Unity of Greater Cleveland. Besides my husband, she was the first person I met involved in New Thought, and she administered my first experience of spiritual healing. During our visit she passed her hands above my body (a technique similar to Qi Gong and Reiki). As she did this she blessed and prayed. Even though she didn't touch me, I distinctly felt the healing warmth of her hands.

Chapter 21

[185]Though specific details may be different, I recognize and thrill to the mystical experiences of many others. Certain factors seem always to be present; there is an all-consuming awareness of being in the Very Presence of the Very God; there is a feeling of bliss, ecstasy, beatitude; there is a conscious knowledge of immortality; and there

is an unquestioned realization that the universe is perfect. I believe that mystical experiences are not as rare as would be suggested by the renown of those that report them. Yet, just as I recognize the essential similarity of my experience with mystical experiences of others, I have also become skeptical of some accounts of mystical revelation. With God anything is possible, and I realize that we all have a tendency to project our own experience and our boundaries onto the rest of the world. But I find it hard to believe that God holds someone's ear for hours or days at a time offering long disquisitions about the minutiae of life—what to eat or what to wear—or that God gives instruction on the conduct of war, or that God spells out the processes of ritual observances or establishes social class structures. In the light of my own experience, I have imaginatively recreated Moses' revelation of the Most High—an experience so earth-shaking that it forced Moses to construct a new worldview in which the nature of humanity and its relationship with God became utterly changed. It goes something like this: I imagine that God's words to Moses were similar to the words I heard: "I am the Lord, your God." From the appearance of God as a burning light and those few words, Moses extrapolated a system that seemed necessarily to follow: "God has spoken to me," Moses might have thought, "and He said He is One: 'I am the Lord.' Why then should I waste my thoughts upon, let alone worship, any false god? And he said 'Your God.' Surely he could not have meant only me, but all my people. 'I Am God' implies a commandment: 'You shall have no other God except me.' Now what does it mean to have no God but 'I Am'? How do we have no other, and how do we prove that we have no other?" Moses proved it in the same way that, hundreds of years later, Jesus' followers proved their faith in Jesus—by their behavior. Jesus' followers asked him how the world would know they belonged to him, seeing that they wore no distinguishing clothing or insignia. Jesus answered, "They will know because ye love one another." Just so, Moses might have thought, "They will know we belong to the One God because we will answer to Him for our actions." And what does it mean to answer to God for your actions? It means to take responsibility for the conduct of your life. In short, Moses concluded that belonging to the One God meant to live not by the rule of accident or destiny, but by rules of righteousness. The whole of the Mosaic Law, the Torah, and the Talmud flow from the effort of the Jews to answer to God for their actions. Judaism is a playing out in history of the first revelation of God to Abraham and the second revelation of God to Moses. By Jesus' time, the Judaism of Moses had become ritualized and mechanized. I believe it was Jesus' mission to return Judaism to its Mosaic purity.

bibliography

Assagioli, Roberto. *Psychosynthesis: A Manual of Principles and Techniques.* New York: Hobbs, Dorman, 1965.

"Art of Aging." *Psychology Today* (January 1984) 32-41.

Benson, Dr. Herbert. *The Mind/Body Effect.* New York: Simon and Schuster, 1979.

———.*Timeless Healing: The Power and Biology of Belief.* New York: Simon and Schuster Audio, 1996.

———.*The Relaxation Response.* New York: Avon, 1975.

Bentov, Itzhak. *Stalking the Wild Pendulum: On the Mechanics of Consciousness.* New York: E.P. Dutton, 1977.

Bloomfield, Harold H., M.D., and Kory, Robert, et al. *Happiness: The TM Program Meditation.* Boston: G.K. Hall, 1976.

Bootzin, Richard R. "The Role of Expectancy in Behavior Change." *Placebo: Theory, Research, and Mechanisms.* Ed. White, Leonard, et al. New York: Guilford Press, 1985.

Borkovec, T.D. "Placebo: Defining the Unknown." *Placebo: Theory, Research, and Mechanisms.* Ed. White, Leonard, et al. New York: Guilford Press, 1985.

Bradshaw, John. *Family Secrets.* New York: Bantam Doubleday Dell Audio, 1995.

Bro, Harmon H., Ph.D. *Edgar Cayce on Dreams.* New York: Warner Books, 1968.

Brody, Howard, M.D. *Placebos and the Philosophy of Medicine.* Chicago: University of Chicago Press, 1980.

———."Placebo Effect: An Examination of Grunbaum's Definition." *Placebo: Theory, Research, and Mechanisms.*

Ed. White, Leonard, et al. New York: Guilford Press, 1985.

Brown, Norman O. *Life Against Death.* New York: Vintage, 1959.

Bucke, Maurice, M.D. *Cosmic Consciousness.* New York: E.P. Dutton, 1923.

Butterworth, Eric. *In the Flow of Life.* New York: Harper & Row, 1975.

———.*Life Is for Loving.* New York: Harper & Row, 1973.

Cady, Emilie, H. *Lessons in Truth.* Unity Village: Unity Books.

Campbell, Joseph. *The Masks of God.* New York: Viking, 1964.

Carter, Mary Ellen. *Edgar Cayce on Prophecy.* New York: Warner Books, 1968.

Cavendish, Richard. *Man, Myth, and Magic: An Illustrated Encyclopedia of the Supernatural.* New York: Marshall Cavendish Corp., 1970.

Chin, Richard M., M.D. *The Energy Within.* New York: Paragon House, 1992.

Chopra, Deepak. *Ageless Body, Timeless Mind.* New York: Harmony, 1993.

———.*Quantum Healing.* New York: Mystic Fire Audio, 1990.

Christian Science Publishing Society. *A Century of Christian Science Healing.* Boston, 1966.

Cousins, Norman. *Anatomy of an Illness.* New York: Norton, 1979.

Curtis, Donald. *Your Thoughts Can Change Your Life.* No. Hollywood: Wilshire Books, 1979.

Dawson, George. *Healing: Pagan and Christian.* New York: AMS Press, Inc., 1977.

DeWitt, John. *The Christian Science Way of Life.* The Christian Science Publishing Co.

Divett, Robert T. *Medicine and the Mormons.* Utah: Horizon, 1981.

Dobbin, Muriel. "When a State Takes Aim at Faith Healing." *US News & World Report* (March 24, 1986).

Dossey, Larry, M.D. *Recovering the Soul.* Bantam Doubleday Dell Audio, 1989.

———.*Reinventing Medicine.* San Francisco: Harper San Francisco, 1999.

Eckhart, Meister.*The Essential Sermons, Commentaries, Treatises, and Defense.* Classics of Western Spirituality. New York: Paulist Press, 1981.

Eddy, Mary Baker. *Science and Health with a Key to the Scriptures.* Boston: The First Church of Christ, Scientist, 1934.

Edmunds, L. Francis. *Rudolph Steiner Education.* Sussex, England:1956.

Ellis, Albert, Ph.D., and Harper, Robert A., Ph.D. *A New Guide to Rational Living.* North Hollywood: Wilshire Book Company, 1975.

Epstein, Mark, M.D. *Thoughts Without a Thinker.* New York: Basic Books, 1995.

Erickson, Milton H., M.D. *My Voice Will Go With You.* New York: W.W. Norton.

Fay, Martha. "A Charmed Circle of Survivors." *Life* (November 1980).

Feigl, Herbert, and Brodbeck, May, eds. *Readings in the Philosophy of Science.* New York: Appleton-Century-Crofts, 1953.

Feldenkrais, Moshe. *Awareness Through Movement.* New York: Harper & Row, 1972.

Ferguson, Marilyn. *The Aquarian Conspiracy.* Los Angeles: Tarcher, 1980.

Ferris, Timothy. *The Mind's Sky.* Beverly Hills: Dove Audio, 1995.

——.*Human Intelligence in a Cosmic Context.* New York: Bantam Books Audio, 1992.

Frank, Jerome, D. *Persuasion and Healing.* 3rd ed. Baltimore: Johns Hopkins University Press, 1991.

Frankl, Viktor E. *Man's Search for Meaning: An introduction to Logotheraphy.* New York: Beacon Press, 1959.

Freeman, James Dillet. *The Story of Unity.* 2nd rev. ed. Unity Village: Unity Books.

Frohock, Fred M. *Healing Powers: Alternative Medicine, Spiritual Communities, and the State.* Chicago: University of Chicago Press, 1992.

Goldsmith, Joel S. *Beyond Words and Thoughts.* Secaucus, N.J.: Citadel Press, 1968.

——.*Conscious Union with God.* Secaucus, N.J.: Citadel Press, 1962.

Gottschalk, Stephen. *The Emergence of Christian Science in American Religious Life.* Berkeley: University of California Press, 1973.

Grunbaum, Adolf. "Explication and Implications of the Placebo Concept." *Placebo: Theory, Research, and Mechanisms.* Ed. White, Leonard, et al. New York: Guilford, 1985.

Hahn, Robert A. "A Sociocultural Model of Illness and Healing." *Placebo: Theory, Research, and Mechanisms.* Ed. White, Leonard, et al. New York: Guilford Press, 1985.

Harpur, Tom. *The Uncommon Touch: An Investigation of Spiritual Healing.* Toronto: McClelland & Stuart, 1994.

Heany, Robert P. "What Choice Did He Have?"*America* (November 22, 1986).

Henig, R.J. "The Placebo Effect: It's Not All in Your Mind." *Sci Quest* (May-June1981):16-20.

Holmes, Ernest. *Seminar Lectures.* Rev. Los Angeles: Science of Mind, 1980.

Holy Bible, Revised Standard Version. New York: Thomas Nelson & Sons, 1952.

Hopkins, Emma Curtis. *High Mysticism.* Marina del Rey, Ca: DeVorss & Co, 1987.

Houston, Jean. *Life Force: The Psycho-Historical Recovery of the Self.* New York: Dell, 1980.

———.*The Possible Human.* Los Angeles: Tarcher,1982.

Hubbard, Roberta. "Gift of the Spirit." *CWRU Magazine* (May 1995).

Huxley, Aldous. *The Doors of Perception.* New York: Harper & Row, 1959.

Illich, Ivan. *Limits to Medicine.* London: McClelland and Steward Limited in association with Marin Boyars, 1976.

———.*Ivan Illich in Conversation.* Interviewed by David Cayley. Anansi,1992.

———.*Medical Nemesis.* New York: Pantheon, 1976.

James, William, *Varieties of Religious Experience.* New York: New American Library, 1958.

Janiger, Oscar, M.D. *A Different Kind of Healing.* New York: Tarcher/Putnam, 1993.

Jaroff, Leon. "Can Attitudes Affect Cancer." *Time* (June 24, 1985):69.

Jerome, Lawrence. *Crystal Power: The Ultimate Placebo Effect.* Buffalo: Prometheus, 1989.

Joy, Brugh, M.D. *Joy's Way.* Los Angeles: J.P. Tarcher, 1979.

Keleman, Stanley. *Your Body Speaks Its Mind.* New York: Simon and Schuster, 1975.

Key, Wilson Bryan. *Subliminal Seduction*. New York: New American Library, 1974.

Keyes, Ken, Jr. *The Hundredth Monkey*. St. Mary: Vision Books, 1982.

Kiev, Ari. *Transcultural Psychiatry*. London: Penguin Books, 1972.

Korzybski, Alfred. *Manhood of Humanity*. 2nd ed. Lakeville, Ct: International Non-Aristotelian Library, 1950.

Krupat, Edward. "A Delicate Imbalance." *Psychology Today* (November 1986):22-26.

Kurtz, Ron and Prestera, Hector, M.D. *The Body Reveals*. San Francisco: Harper & Row, 1976.

Laing, R.D. *Knots*. New York: Vintage,1970.

Levine, Jon D. and Gordon, Newton C. "Growing Pains in Psychobiological Research." *Placebo: Theory, Research, and Mechanisms*. Ed. White, Leonard, et al. New York: Guilford Press, 1985.

Lynn, Steven Jay, and Rhue, Judith W. "Daydream Believers." *Psychology Today* (September 1985):22-36.

Maimonides. *The Book of Knowledge from the Mishneh Torah of Maimonides*. Trans. Russell, H.M., and Weinberg, Rabbi J. New York: Ktav, 1983.

Maltz, Maxwell, M.D. *Psycho-Cybernetics and Self-fulfillment*. New York: Bantam, 1973.

———.*Psycho-Cybernetics*. Englewood Cliffs: Prentice-Hall, Inc., 1960.

Matt, Daniel C. *The Essential Kabbalah*. San Francisco: Harper San Francisco, 1996.

Mazzolini, Joan, and David, Dave. "Bad Law Behind Bad Medicine." *Cleveland Plain Dealer,* Sunday Magazine (June 12, 1993):18-A.

McLuhan, Marshall, and Fiore, Quentin. *The Medium Is*

the Message. New York: Bantam, 1967.

———.Understanding Media. 2nd ed. New York: New American Library, 1964.

Moss, Richard, M.D. The Black Butterfly: An Invitation to Radical Aliveness. Berkeley: Celestial Arts, 1986.

Needleman, Jacob. The New Religions. New York: Crossroad, 1984.

Ornish, Dean, M.D. Eat More, Weigh Less. New York: HarperCollins, 1993.

Ornstein, Robert E., ed. The Nature of Human Consciousness. New York: Viking, 1974.

Ouspensky, P.D. The Fourth Way. New York: Vintage, 1971.

Peel, Robert. Spiritual Healing in a Scientific Age. New York: Harper & Row, 1987.

Perls, Frederick. Gestalt Therapy Verbatim. Highland, NJ: Center for Gestalt Development, 1988.

Plotkin, William B. "A Psychological Approach to Placebo: The Role of Faith in Therapy and Treatment." Placebo: Theory, Research, and Mechanisms. Ed. White, Leonard, et al. New York: Guilford Press, 1985.

Podmore, Frank. From Mesmer to Christian Science. New York: New York University, 1909.

Rajneesh, Bhagwan Shree. Meditation: The Art of Ecstasy. New York: Harper & Row, 1976.

Rawllinson, Mary Crenshaw. "Truth Telling and Paternalism in the Clinic: Philosophical Reflectins on the Use of Placebos in Medical Practice." Placebo: Theory, Research, and Mechanisms. Ed. White, Leonard, et al. New York: Guilford Press, 1985.

Ray, Sondra. Loving Relationships. Berkeley: Celestial Arts, 1995.

Reich, Wilhelm. The Function of the Orgasm. New York:

Farrar, Straus, and Giroux, 1973.

Rhinehart, Luke. *The Book of EST*. New York: Holt, Rinehart and Winston, 1976.

Robinsom, Wheeler, H. *The Old Testament: Its Making and Meaning*. New York: Abington Press, 1937.

Rogers, Carl, and Stevens, Barry. *Person to Person*. New York: Pocket Books, 1971.

Russell, H.M., Weinberg, J, trans. *The Book of Knowledge from the Mishneh Torah of Maimonides*. New York: Ktav Publishing House, Inc., 1983.

Sapir, Edward. *Culture, Language, and Personality*. Los Angeles: Univ. of California Press, 1957.

Sheldrake, Rupert. *The Presence of the Past*. New York: Vintage, 1989.

Shullins, Nancy. "Trauma Leaves Bilogical Clues," *Cleveland Plain Dealer* (1996):1-j.

Skrabanek, Petr, Ph.D, and McCormick, James, M.D. *Follies and Fallacies in Medicine*. Buffalo: Prometheus Books, 1990.

St. Leger, A.S., and Cochrane, Al. "The Anomaly that Wouldn't Go Away." *Lancet 2* (1978):1153.

Troward, Thomas. *The Edinburgh Lectures on Mental Science*. New York: Roger Brothers, 1909.

Trungpa, Chogyam. *Buddhism and Meditation*. Big Sur Recording, 1989.

Ukens, Carol. "The Tragic Truth." *Drug Topics* (November 6, 1995):66-67.

Viscott, David. *Emotional Resilience*. Abridged. New York: Random House Audiobooks, 1996.

———.*Risking*. Los Angeles: Audio Renaissance Tapes, 1989.

Watts, Alan W. "The World Series" Audio lectures. Sausalito, Calif.: MEA.

——.*The Two Hands of God.* New York: George Braziller, 1963.

——.*The Way of Zen.* New York: Vintage, 1957.

White, Leonard; Tursky, Bernard; Schwartz, Gary E., eds. *Placebo: Theory, Research, and Mechanisms.* New York: Guilford Press, 1985.

——."Proposed Synthesis of Placebo Models." *Placebo: Theory, Research, and Mechanisms.* Ed. White, Leonard, et al. New York: Guilford Press, 1985.

Williamson, Marianne. *A Return to Love.* New York: HarperCollins, 1992.

——.*A Woman's Worth.* Abridged. New York: Random House Audio Books, 1993.

Worchester, Elwood, and McComb, Samuel. *Body, Mind, and Spirit.* Boston: Marshall Jones, 1931.

Yee, Laura. "Homeopathic Remedies Can Work." *The Cleveland Plain Dealer* (17 April, 1994):4H.

Zukav, Gary. *The Dancing Wu Li Masters:* An Overview of the New Physics. New York: William Morrow & Co, 1979.

——.*The Seat of the Soul.* New York: Simon & Schuster, 1989.

Please send the stories of your experiences to:

Mystical Experiences of Ordinary People
c/o Warwick Associates
18340 Sonoma Highway
Sonoma, CA 95476